Blessings of the Blood: A Book of Menstrual Lore and Rituals for Women

Rituals, Volume 1

Celu Amberstone

Published by Kashallan Press, 2022.

BLESSINGS OF THE BLOOD: A BOOK OF MENSTRUAL LORE AND RITUALS FOR WOMEN

First edition. June 30, 2022.

Copyright © 2022 Celu Amberstone.

ISBN: 978-1990581038

Written by Celu Amberstone.

Table of Contents

This book is dedicated to our daughters everywhere.

In the past twenty some years women have asked me to reissue this book and finally with the help of my dear friend Paula Johanson and her daughter, it is finally happening. This new edition of Blessings of the Blood is dedicated to my daughter Karlynn Walker and my granddaughters Tuuli, Aurora and Xyla, as well as the many adopted daughters I have been blessed to know over the years, Dianne, Kathy, Sky, Michelle and so many more. This book is my gift to you and the future generations of women who will be searching for their power. Once again I would like to thank the many women who shared with me their stories for the original edition and the few new contributors to this one.

With love and Blessings,

Cornwoman (Celu Amberstone)

Menstruation is a difficult topic for many women to talk about without feeling vulnerable. For this reason, I have changed some of my informants' initials, or the location where they live, to protect their privacy. Any resemblance to women who were not contributors is purely coincidental.

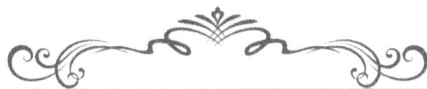

Preface

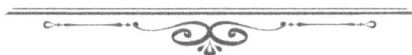

This book grew out of my own spiritual quest to find a deeper meaning to my bodily cycles. Unfortunately, it is not easy to find a positive image of menstruation. If you ask most women about their period they will probably tell you it is either a curse or a nuisance. During my search I reviewed countless books on the Premenstrual Syndrome, and texts that psychoanalyzed my monthly flow, but very few of the works I read offered women a positive image of menstruation or told women that through their monthly Bleeding spiritual growth and healing could be attained. In the area of women's spirituality there are books that have fragments of this ancient knowledge, but nowhere could I find a book written by women, for women, that brought together the fragments of ancient and modern menstrual lore.

As I became more and more frustrated I decided there was only one thing I could do – create the type of book I was looking for by myself. I began simply by asking friends and acquaintances for ideas and information on this subject. After some initial hesitation, I found almost every woman I talked to had something to share. I became fascinated by my growing collection of notes and stories.

As I collected information, I also began to share it with other women in my classes and workshops. I found this to be a mixed blessing. Many women were extremely positive and supportive of my work, while at other times, in the most unexpected places, my project was met with extreme fear and hostility. It became very clear to me that most of us, no matter how liberated we may think we are, still harbour deep fear and hostility towards our monthly cycle.

After about a year I had a number of tragic stories in which women expressed the pain and fear they experience around their periods; I also had information on herbal and folk remedies for these ills. Except for my

3

own intuitive writing, however, I had little content that expressed a spiritual aspect of the menstrual cycle.

Through my own prayers and meditations I had begun to feel a sense of joy and celebration about my cycle and I wanted to share that with other women – especially younger women – in hopes that their life's journey would be less fearful than those of my generation. What are the rituals of first Blood that should mark our passage into womanhood, and what are the rituals of last Blood to honour and celebrate the wisdom of our Elders? Alas, they are sadly missing from most of our lives.

It's not good enough to read about such rites in the sterile pages of anthropology books. They must become a real and vibrant part of our lives today. I knew that within the growing world-wide pagan community other women were feeling the same need I was, so I sent out a letter to many Wiccan and pagan publications asking for women's input for my proposed book.

I am pleased to say that the response was good. My deepest gratitude goes to all the women who have shared with me and supported this project.

Within these pages, women from a variety of races, ages, cultures, and life-styles tell their stories and pass on the knowledge of their womanhood. Included are first Blood stories, herbal folk remedies for cramps and other health problems, Wiccan Blood rituals, and the wisdom of our grandmothers. [Wicca is the name given to the "old religion," or the Western European shamanic tradition.]

In respecting the desire of many women to maintain their privacy, I have chosen to give a minimum of biographical data about my informants, and refer to them by initials only – except in the case of a few well-known authors and professional women whom the reader may wish to know.

My special thanks to Vicki Noble, Susan Weed, Starhawk, Margot Adler, Brook Medicine Eagle, Rosemary Gladstar and Jean Mountaingrove for taking time from their busy schedules to support this project.

I strongly believe that no matter where we live, or what our lifestyle, we are all of us are bonded together as women by the bond of our menstrual Blood. It is time that we as women reclaim our birthright and give back to our daughters and ourselves a positive, powerful image of womanhood. To that end this book is dedicated to our daughters and the future.

Cornwoman

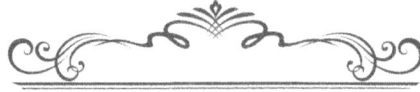

Memories of the Menarche

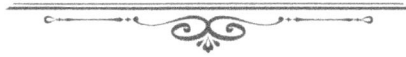

First Blood Stories

I STARTED BLEEDING today
I feel wonderful, so alive
I sit, and look out my window
like a big red rose opening
to the warmth of the sun
I feel so wonderful, so alive
this is my special day.
T.C.

CONSIDERING THE AMOUNT of information and the number of experiences we store in our memories throughout our lives, it is amazing that almost every woman remembers her first menstrual period. No matter whether the event itself was ordinary, exciting, or frightening, the memory is locked in her mind so that even in old age it can still be recalled quite vividly.

These vivid memories, over time, point out the importance of the menarche in a woman's life. For some (the lucky ones), those young girls who are informed and proud of their maturing bodies, the first Blood is an exciting, pleasant time to be savoured and shared with family and friends.

Unfortunately, for all too many women, the menarche is an initiation into confusion, humiliation, and fear. Around the world an atmosphere of ignorance and fear surrounds menstruation in general, and the menarche in particular. There are countless anthropological studies that speak of the horrors of the menarche throughout the ages. It has been the fate of many young girls to have been beaten, mutilated, locked in cages or darkened rooms, or accused of demonic possession at the time of their first Blood.

In these pages are the stories of several women who wish to share their memories of their first Blood. Their experiences are representative of women's experiences from all races and cultural backgrounds throughout the world.

❧

B.C., HOUSEWIFE IN her 40's; Detroit, MI

My first Blood came right on my twelfth birthday. I can remember having very vivid dreams that night but I can't remember exactly what. When I woke up, the bed sheet was covered in blood. I called my mom. She had already told me a little and given me a book to read, so I wasn't frightened. Actually I was quite excited. My mother took me into the bathroom and showed me how to use the belt and napkin. I guess she had been prepared, too, because everything was ready and brand new. I felt very excited and so grown up. Later, my best friend came over. I felt so proud. She asked me how I felt. I felt fine but I said I had a bit of cramps. I don't know where I got the idea that I should have cramps but it seemed like the event was too important not to have something different to say. And cramps, well that's what I'd heard older women complain of, so I said cramps. My dad came up to me later that first day I started. He seemed very embarrassed but he said something (I don't remember what) and gave me a kiss. It was nice, but a bit embarrassing because he was so embarrassed. After the first one, I fell into the routine as regular as clockwork, every thirty days until I reached my forties, when my cycle began to change.

❧

J.R., WAITRESS IN HER 50's; Chicago, IL

My family was sharecroppers in South Carolina when I was a young girl. There was nine of us, my mama and daddy, and us seven children. I was the oldest girl. My mama never told me nothing about the curse before I got it. People who grows up in the city thinks farm children knows everything about sex and such things but it's not true.

Sure I seen animals do it but I never saw anybody except the babies without their clothes on. When I lived in Chicago as a grown woman my roommate used to laugh at me because sometimes when I got up in the morning I'd put my streetclothes on over my pajamas. I was kind of shy to undress in front of people and that's what I'd done at home. Our house was so small and never any privacy; it was sort of a habit I guess.

I was eleven when my periods started and 'cause of how we lived, I didn't know much about my body. As I said, my mama, she never told me anything. I guess she thought I was too young. The day it happened my mama was away. She used to do day work in town sometimes. I was home with the younger children. I'd felt bad all morning but I ignored it because my dad was home sick. He used to drink sometime and he was real mean when he was drinking. I was afraid of him then. So, I was working and trying to keep the babies quiet. I remember I was putting out the clothes and I felt something wet running down my leg. When I seen it was blood I got real scared. I didn't want to tell my dad; I was more scared of him the way he was. Well, I thought I was going to die. I had cramps so bad. I tried to do my work and I was just praying I'd stay alive 'til my mama came home. When she did I ran into her arms sobbing. I was so relieved she was home. I told her I was dying. I was crying so hard I couldn't talk right. Finally she got out of me what was wrong. She looked at me real sad. I'll never forget that. She told me I was a woman now and that I mustn't let any man kiss me or I'd get pregnant and my daddy would throw me out for shaming the family. That was all. We didn't have Kotex out there on the farm so my mama showed me how to use rags. She didn't say much else. It was years later when I went to live with an aunt in Detroit and I started going to school regular that I read some books and learned what it was all about.

◈◈◈

B.B., TEACHER AND MOTHER in her 20's; Vancouver, BC

My family was very private. I never saw their bodies. My mother and older sister always emerged from the bathroom fully groomed and dressed. I remember my older sister trying to talk to me about my period before it happened, but she was always very vague saying things like Did you ever see anything red in your panties? or Someday you might find some blood down there. If you do, tell me or mom. I didn't understand what she was saying so I forgot about it. When it came I was so afraid and humiliated, I locked myself in the bathroom and refused to come out. After a while, my sister came home and tried to get me out of there, but I wouldn't budge. I was going to stay in there until I died. I guess she figured out what was wrong with me and went to get my mom. My mom and aunt were in the bar down the street. They came back loud and a little drunk. They pounded on the bathroom door trying to make me come out, but I wouldn't. They seemed happy telling anyone who would listen that I was a woman now. I was so humiliated. Finally they went back to the bar to celebrate.

Later my sister got me to come out and showed me how to use the belt and pads. After that I was very secretive about my period. I never told anyone when it was, and wrapped my pads very carefully so no one would know.

<hr>

M.T.C., LEGAL SECRETARY in her late 40's; Seattle, WA

I'm thankful to have had the enlightened parents that I did. I realize now that, growing up in the fifties, I was very lucky. My parents were very open about their bodies and sex. When my period came at age thirteen, it was no problem. I had read some books and my mother had talked to me frankly about what was going to happen. I was informed and ready when it came. The day my periods started, my parents took me and a girlfriend out to dinner at a fancy restaurant. I got all dressed up, had my hair done, and was even allowed to wear some make-up. I felt very grown up-like a real lady. I remember my father gave me and my girlfriend (who had already started her periods) each a beautiful corsage. It was a lovely evening. Looking back on it all, I realize that my preparation for womanhood was very advanced for the time but it was also very cold and clinical. Physically I was prepared, but emotionally-well, not so much. My mother still considered menstruation, at best, a nuisance. Something a woman tried to ignore if she could. She was very much an advocate for women's rights and part of being equal with men was pretending that menstruation didn't exist, or at least that it couldn't slow a good woman down.

In the past few years I've been studying Wicca. I realize now that what was missing from my memories was a sense of emotional involvement. I was luckier than most to be taken out to dinner, but I see there is a need to share with our daughters our deeper feeling about our bodies and the special power and magic that can be found in being a Bleeding woman.

H.S., STUDENT IN HER early 30's; Vancouver, BC

I don't remember much about my first period except that my mother gave me a ring that had belonged to her mother. She said it was sort of a family tradition to pass this ring on to the oldest daughter when she had her first period.

My mother told me I was a woman now and that the ring (a ruby set in a plain gold band) was very old and very special. I was to keep it in my jewelry box and never wear it out to play because I might lose it. I was to keep it safe and then pass it on to my own daughter one day. Her trust in me made me feel proud. I still have that ring and when my daughter is old enough I'll pass it on to her.

J.N., MUSIC TEACHER in her late 40's; Victoria, BC

I first menstruated when I was eleven. I had been skipping rope with the girls and I went inside to go to the bathroom. I saw blood and called my mother. She had given me a book to read so I knew what it was. My mother pinned a face-cloth in my pants because she didn't have any pads as she was past menopause (she was fifty-two). I went outside and announced to my friends that I had just started to menstruate and I was a woman now and they were just girls and they could all go home – and they did. (I was beyond skipping rope.)

My mother said we were going to the next town to visit friends. The friends had a daughter, one year younger than me, who had died of leukemia when she was five. I always missed her when I was there and felt alienated, as her mother barely acknowledged my presence. The women were in the house talking. The men were in the garden. I stood at the other end of the garden looking at the fish or pretending to. I wondered if Mr. B. could tell by looking at me that I was menstruating. I began to feel guilty. I felt like peeing. I wondered if that was menstruation. After a great deal of deliberation I decided it was and let it go. I soon realized I'd wet the whole face-cloth and something wasn't right. I went and got my mother. She was really mad at me and asked how I could be so stupid and that she didn't have another face-cloth or pad and Jenny didn't either and we'd have to go right home.

B.W., HOUSEWIFE IN her late 30's; Victoria, BC

I remember, at onset of menses, feeling that this was to be something precious and private. My mom phoned her aunt with the news. I felt betrayed.

J.Z.N., PSYCHIC READER in her 40's; Victoria, BC

My first Bleeding was at the age of twelve. I was absolutely unaware of the process and it came as a great shock to me. I honestly believed I was dying. My mother and I had a very difficult relationship. I suspect part of the reason was that we are quite similar in temperament and I know she has never been very comfortable with who she is.

Anyway, I had come home from school to find that I was definitely in some kind of trouble with her again. (I had developed a strong and intuitive sense about that kind of thing.) As I sat in my room doing my homework and awaiting my doom, I decided to venture forth into the bathroom, stomach madly churning and gnawing because my bladder felt ready to burst.

And there it was – blood in my underwear! "That's it," I thought, "my body can't take this stress anymore and I'm dying!" And from that forbidden zone too! "Mom," I called feebly. She sent my father.

"What's the matter?" His voice was half-hearted.

"I'm bleeding." My voice shook but I was determined to be in control. The next thing I knew the atmosphere changed. Doom was dispersed and replaced with confidentiality. My mother took me into the forbidden sanctuary of her room, hauled out a box of Kotex and this funny looking belt, and gave me some song and dance of which the only part I can remember now is that she said I could get pregnant if I was kissed or touched by boys. It was such a shock because I was totally unprepared. I'd never seen a box of Kotex either at home or in the stores. I had never heard mom or any of her women friends atlk about it. Later it used to bother me that they called it 'menistration.' They couldn't even pronounce the word right.

After my first period nothing happened for months and I really couldn't figure out what was happening. I thought this was supposed to be a regular occurrence. Then I thought that my body had betrayed me again. I felt so alienated from the whole process until years later I was trying to explain my condition delicately to a friend and she said Oh, you're having your period. That was when I realized that other women menstruated and that it was a perfectly natural occurrence.

This type of experience was something that I never wanted to have happen to my girls so I've always been very open with them about things. When my oldest daughter started, we didn't have a ritual, but a friend and I took both of our daughters out for an elegant dinner and discussed elegant things like career paths and their changing bodies. For me it was a real turning point in my relationship with my daughter. Though it was very subtle, I felt she had come into her own then. I'm still there for her but our relationship is very different now. It is like there is another woman in the house, and I have loved that transition.

❧

A BLOOD WORKSHOP; VICTORIA, BC

I remember a time, it must be nineteen years ago now (and I still feel the embarrassment). I was fifteen or sixteen and knew nothing. Growing up in England, menstruation was referred to as the curse, a term I never questioned. There was no mystery or power – just the unmentionable.

I've never talked of this incident before. I was an exchange student in Germany and I did not know how to dispose of my napkins. I would have been painfully embarrassed to ask in English, never mind German! So they stayed in my closet. They began to smell and my host mother finally had to broach the subject to me and remove them. That sounds, as I write it, like a story from medieval Europe, not the twentieth century. I still blush to remember.

⚜

M., SECRETARY IN HER 30's; Nanaimo, BC

When I was twelve, I awoke one morning in a bed that felt warm and wet. I thought I had wet the bed and was overwhelmed with shame. I pushed back the covers and found that the bed was soaked with blood. I was terrified. Not daring to move in case all my insides fell out, I screamed for my mother. That was my introduction to the curse.

On no account was my father or brother to see anything, or to suspect that I was menstruating. Paper parcels were smuggled furtively out of the bathroom.

⚜

V., FARMER IN HER 40'S; Aldergrove, BC

My first period – my mother tried to make me feel special and grown-up, but because we had never talked of it before, the subject seemed an alienating one.

⚜

S.D., FARMER IN HER 40's; Aldergrove, BC

My first period was horrendous. I was ten years old and I had no idea what was happening. I thought I must have cut myself somehow and kept trying to put band-aids on. Finally, my mother noticed bloody toilet paper in the bathroom, called me in, and asked me if I had the Curse, but I didn't know what it was. She showed me her sanitary napkins and her belt and told me how to use them; she also told me that I could borrow her belt. I asked her why she wasn't using it – thinking I was now going to bleed for the rest of my life.

⚜

L.H., TRAPPER IN HER 40's; Alaska

Before my old granny died, she once told me that, when she was a young girl, our people had special ceremonies for a girl when she started her periods. They used to build a little lodge for her out in the bush, but not too far from camp. Inside was everything she would need for several months stay. During this time a girl would stay alone. She would have to set rabbit snares, catch fish, do everything for herself. Maybe one of the old women would come and check on her from time to time and teach her things, but mostly she was alone. When it was time, she would be brought back to camp and they would have a feast. From then on, that girl would be thought of as a woman, and her family would probably arrange a marriage for her not long after. That was how it was for us here in the North back then.

⸎

P., UNIVERSITY STUDENT in her early 20's; Victoria, BC

My period started when I was on my dad's sailboat. I had been conceived on a sailboat so having my period come while on another boat seemed special to me. I thought I would be embarrassed with my dad there because he and my mom were divorced, but it turned out okay. My dad's new wife had what I needed on board. I didn't feel embarrassed at all. I felt soft and beautiful, with no discomfort. I have good memories of my first Blood with the wind and the sea rocking me to sleep.

⸎

A.D., COMPUTER PROGRAMMER in her 30's; Calgary, AB

I used to masturbate at night in my bed. My mother had warned me about touching myself "down there," so wouldn't you know I started menstruating when I was asleep. I woke up and felt all sticky. I put my finger down there and saw blood. I was so frightened. First I thought I had really injured myself this time, and I might even die. I stayed there a long time not knowing what to do. I didn't feel too bad, but I was sure my mother would find out I'd been playing with myself again and I'd catch it for sure. I tried to keep from telling her as long as I could, hoping it would go away, but it didn't. I finally had to tell her and to my surprise she didn't even ask me if I had been masturbating again. She just took me to the bath and showed me how to use the stuff and that was that. I learned more later from my friends at school which was a great relief.

❦

A.L., PHYSIOTHERAPIST in her late 20's; Tacoma, WA

At best I can remember, my close friends and I all knew about menstruation months before any of us got it. We had seen a movie at school and occasionally talked about it and what it would be like. I remember us taking bets as to who would get it first and sneaking into the drugstore to check out the Kotex display. If the male clerks noticed us, we would run outside giggling.

Judy was the first in my circle to have her period. We were all very jealous. She lorded it over us for a while but we didn't care because we were all so excited and curious. We plied her with questions until Margaret got hers three weeks later. I was one of the last to start. I can remember feeling so left out that I even prayed to God to kind of help me and make it start soon. Later, I couldn't understand why I had been in such a hurry because sometimes menstruation can be a real nuisance.

❦

D.N., UNIVERSITY STUDENT in her 20's; Montreal, QC

I learned about menstruation from the man who was sexually molesting me from age eleven to thirteen. He kept me well informed on what I should expect from my body. My mother never told me anything. He told me my periods would hurt a lot but I didn't believe him because deep down I knew it didn't have to hurt and it never has.

❦

N.B., WAITRESS IN HER 30's; Edmonton, AB

I had a very embarrassing experience during my first period. When it first happened, my mother instructed me in the use of belt and pads and told me to wrap my napkins up carefully and put them in the trash. I did just as she had said but the next day my dad found one of my pads on the bathroom floor. My mother confronted me about it and we argued. I ended up in tears because I knew I had done as she had said. Later, I saw the dog take another pad out of the garbage. It had been him that made the mess. Then I realized I had to take my pads to the kitchen garbage where he couldn't reach them. Later I told my mom. She sort of apologized but I still felt awful that my dad and probably my older brothers had seen my bloody pads on the floor.

⁘

M.A., AUTHOR; NEW YORK, NY

When I got my first period, I was at a friend's house, staying overnight. I knew what it was, since my mother had had a long talk with me, but it was still strange to suddenly see it there. My friend's mother got all the stuff I needed and then poured me a glass of wine and toasted my womanhood. I will never forget how wonderful I felt when the whole family toasted me. I have always wondered whether the fact that I almost never have cramps, depression, etc. has to do with the fact that this part of my life was celebrated as a gift from the beginning.

⁘

S., WITCH IN HER 50'S; San Francisco, CA

My fourteen-year-old granddaughter told me that she felt she was psychic just before her period began. I explained to her that she probably was – that this was a time of "power" for women. I was surprised to hear her story because there isn't anything in her family environment that would teach her woman-spiritual ways. My pagan thoughts and ways are entirely my own and private.

⁘

C.N.S., TEACHER IN her late 40's; Victoria, BC

Each year, during my teaching career in Home Economics, I set aside a time for a series of talks, slides, and discussions with my students about the development of their bodies, menstruation, and attitudes. Of all my experiences related to this exchange, one stands out as the most powerful.

A Native Indian girl came to me after class to tell me how thankful she was that we had talked about periods as no one had shared anything about these changes with her and she actually thought she was going to die. When she shared this with me, I hugged her and told her she could always come to me to talk about anything she wished. The powerful feelings I have about a young girl having to experience such pain and terror with no one to talk to still moves me to tears.

⁊⁊⁊

M., TEACHER IN HER 30's; Victoria, BC

My period started when I was eleven. I don't remember the date except that it was summer and very hot. We had gone out on a school trip to a safari park near Liverpool to mark our "passage" from junior to secondary school. It was very exciting. I felt nothing amiss except, on the way back in the confines of the coach, the discomfort of being hot and kind of sticky. I remember especially feeling damp between my legs – sweaty I thought – and the dampness made my legs rub and feel uncomfortable.

When I got home my mum and I had to prepare to go out again to see my older sister in a play. As usual, I was very chatty and excited; we were in the bathroom, my mum putting cream on her face, me having a pee.

Then the Blood. Not much, but definitely red, definitely "there." I was shocked, silenced, dumbfounded. Whose could it be but mine? Instinctively I knew it was, but the realization numbed me. I wasn't afraid, as such, but I was appalled. Then my mum saw and was a bit shocked too, I think, but she was actually quite calm and matter of fact when she said it's your period or something like that. So I knew the Blood was normal. I had heard of periods, though I didn't really know what they were supposed to be, except that Blood was somehow involved and they were supposed to come "later on." I hadn't expected it to be so soon. I knew I didn't want it.

I knew my older sister had "started" and that it had, ever so slightly and in an undefinable way, changed things. All I knew was that it somehow made life different. It made it so that things had to be hidden and secret (even from me though we had always been close). My mother and sister would confer in hushed tones and then disappear into the other room where mysterious things were done, things surrounded by unmentionables and, for me, unimaginables. I didn't want to have any part of that. It went against the grain of my being. It wasn't me.

But now here was the Blood, dooming me. I grasped that from now on I too would have to hide and conceal. I knew I would have to ensure that no one knew. After all, I had never seen anything from either my mum or sister; and before my sister had started her period, I had no inclination of anything at all. It had obviously been a well kept secret. Did that mean it was something to be ashamed of if you had to hide it so? Was I supposed to feel shame for this, though it was something I had no control over, something that just "happened"? I suddenly felt incredibly burdened, powerless, faced with the coming of this Blood.

When my mum brought out the belt and pad and showed me how to use it, I resigned myself to putting it on, still too numb to say anything. I remember that, while putting it on, I felt defeated and humiliated. The one thing I asked my mum was not what it was, though I had no idea of the "meaning'" of this Blood (and didn't until much later), but how long it would last. She explained that a woman would Bleed like this every month until she was forty-five or so, then she would stop. I felt a distinct sinking feeling; I was trapped, caught for the rest of my life. At the same time, almost unconsciously, I picked up my mother's reference to "woman." Was I a woman, I wondered? I certainly wasn't considered one. And my mum didn't suggest that because I was Bleeding I was a woman. In fact she and my sister discussed precisely how incapable and "messy" they thought I'd be in dealing with this. I could also feel childhood slipping away. I felt robbed somehow; this Blood was going to lose me my freedom and I felt the pain of loss in me.

CRONE CIRCLE WOMEN, women in their 50's and 60's;
Victoria, BC
1.
I started my periods very late, and my mother was very worried and beginning to wonder if I was doing something. I didn't start menstruating until I was fifteen. I was very happy when my periods started. I wasn't told anything by her. I was just given a book to read.

2.

I think I got the same book and a box of Kotex in the cupboard. I remember that day quite vividly because there was Blood! Later I went in and told mom I was Bleeding and she said '"Well, I put the box in your cupboard, dear." I do remember she let me stay home from school that day and lie on her bed with cushions. I was fourteen, and this was such a treat to be in my mother's bed. It felt kind of special.

3.

I wanted to have my period because I went to a little one room school where I knew a lot about the other students and I did want to feel grown up. However, I caught the measles at the end of my sophomore year. I was very sick and at the end of that time I got my period. This was also around the time of the fall of Dunkirk in World War II. It was a chaotic time for me and all the world. Being very sick, all I could do was listen to the radio. I felt terrible. Now it seems so symbolic. Those were bloody, bloody times, and then my own Blood coming.

4.

I remember being allowed to stay home that day but it wasn't a happy day because my mother said "Oh, you poor thing. You've finally begun the curse." I was fourteen. I remember it as a very painful, unhappy day. I had the feeling that I had done something terrible to bring this on myself, and I think a lot of guilt began for me then.

5.

I was very late when I started. I was sixteen, coming up seventeen. I remember the girls at school being able to get out of gym when they had their periods. I learned what a privilege that was so the first thing I did when I got my period was go to the gym teacher and tell her I couldn't take gym that day because I had my period. I had the most healthy periods so there was no reason for me not to take gym. I didn't suffer with them at all, but I was bound and determined I was going to get off like the other girls did. The other thing I remember was that I started shaving my legs before I started menstruating. While learning to shave my legs I cut myself and my sister saw the blood on the sheets. She was so envious because she thought I'd gotten my period.

❦

J.N., MUSIC TEACHER in her late 40's; Victoria, BC

I remember, around the time of my first period, my mother took me aside and told me that, when I went to the drugstore to buy pads, to check the drugstore out to make sure there was a female clerk. She would buy them for me the first time but after that I would have to get my own. One time, when I was fifteen or sixteen, I went into the drugstore and the female clerk wasn't around yet; just the druggist was there. Since it wasn't an embarrassment to buy pads anymore, I decided to get them from the druggist. I don't think he was embarrassed about selling pads to me but was uncomfortable because I was so embarrassed. However, that was kind of a break-through. After that, I have not been at all shy about buying pads anywhere.

❦

H.S., PSYCHOLOGIST in her 30's; Los Angeles, CA

I have no memory, positive or negative, of my first Blood flow. My family was quite open about bodily functions and my mother was quite uninhibited and sensual. I'm sure I was fully informed about menstruation long before my Blood flow, and that I perceived it as very natural. Though I began my Blood flow at age ten or so, I never experienced cramps until I was sixteen. My mother was very sympathetic and showed me yoga and breathing exercises to ease my discomfort.

We also talked about the possibility of emotional stress triggering the cramps since this was not a usual occurrence for me. Although I have only kept track of my cycle in recent years (I'm thirty-two now) and I was very irregular in my cycle until my mid-twenties, I always intuited when my Blood flow was starting and always went to the bathroom in the first few moments. I took a kind of secret pride in this attunement to my body.

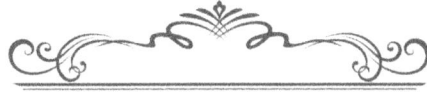

Rituals of First Blood

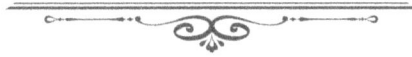

from Mother to Daughter

THE BLOOD-LINE
> *Passes from one mother*
> *To the next.*
> *We carry our mothers*
> *Within. Without.*
> *The Blood-line is wet.*
> *K.P.*

THE RITUALS GIVEN IN this chapter are meant to be used as guidelines for women wishing to create first Blood rites for their daughters or themselves. They are not necessarily meant to be copied exactly as they are written. These are just a few of the many possibilities.

Though it may appear to many women that we have lost almost all of our ancient tradition, this is true only of the surface reality. Deep down, in our cells, in our DNA, ancient memories still exist. We still know all that we need to know. We need only take the time to remember.

I am always saddened when I hear other people say how lucky I am to be a Native because I have such a rich cultural tradition to guide me. I am glad for the gift of my tradition, but, as I grow older, I see more and more clearly its strengths and weaknesses. Strong traditions can become binding prisons when the form of a tradition is rigidly held on to while the meaning behind the tradition is long forgotten. As we approach a new age, all of us need to learn from each other. There is no one group that has a monopoly

21

on the way. New rituals must be created by adapting our traditions to meet and reflect our world today. In other words, the form of a ritual can change over the years as long as the spirit of that rite remains clear and unchanged. As women, we have forgotten a lot of our ancient knowledge. It is possible to reclaim our past and build on it for the future. With patience and love, and by drawing on the principles of ritual that have survived, we can create for ourselves and our children a meaningful way of life.

STARHAWK, AUTHOR AND witch; San Francisco, CA

One thing that can be done for a first Blood ritual is to make a special garment for the young woman. P. made her daughter a robe but she later grew out of it. Now a friend is preparing for her oldest daughter who will be having her first period soon. She decided to make her a cloak and to make it with a detachable hood so that her daughter would have two hoods; she planned to embroider designs on one hood (her ritual hood) and then she could make a plain hood so that her daughter could wear the cape as a regular cloak. She could wear it anytime she wanted, for rituals in general as well as for her period. Another garment often used is a red scarf or a red belt. You must prepare the child for the ritual by discussing it in detail with her. Some girls allow it to be done because they know it is important for their mother's women's group, although at the time it may not be a big deal to them. Later, they will look back and understand, and it will really mean something to them.

V., FARMER IN HER 40'S; Aldergrove, BC

I have been looking around here and there for information on first Blood rituals. My daughter is just turning ten and I want to be able to give her a sense of power as a woman and to let her join with us in our women's circle for a celebration at that time. I feel very fortunate that we have our group to welcome her, but we are in a situation where we will basically be making up our own rituals. The feast part will be easy – some succulent red fruit

– pomegranate seems appropriate, bowls of cherries (carve the pits into a necklace?).

There is no limit to what can be imagined, although I feel that there is such a void to operate in; no tradition to hand on from mother to daughter. We must create these new rituals wisely and give them lovingly so our daughters will take them as givers and pass them on.

I would dearly love my daughter to truly celebrate this time in her life. One way we are going to mark it is by getting her ears pierced (something she wants to do, but is enjoying saving for the occasion). I really want our women's group to have some kind of ritual prepared to welcome her into the circle. There is another woman, with a child the same age, who feels the same way.

I know that I would like my daughter to save her first Blood as there would be so much power involved in it. I can see some kind of amulet being created to carry the dried Blood. My fear is that, in sharing her knowledge with her peers, she will be singled out as some kind of weirdo. I don't know how to prevent or deal with that, I just want to protect her from having to deal with that kind of energy. Our women's group is strong and hopefully will provide the necessary counterbalance.

⚜

S.D., FARMER IN HER 40's; Aldergrove, BC

I was new to the craft when my daughter started menstruating four years ago. Some of my friends were here on her first Blood and we tried to whip up a celebration, which she refused to come to. I'm proud that she refused, although I was sad at the time. I probably needed to mark the transition, so we did the ritual without her.

I hope my daughter has a better understanding of the physical part of her menstrual cycle, but I'm not sure how successful I was in mothering her. It's still an area she prefers not to discuss. I try to respect her need for privacy, but there are still times when I embarrass her with my indiscretions, like discussing what brand of sanitary napkins we prefer.

⚜

J.Z.N., PSYCHIC READER in her 40's; Victoria, BC

When my eldest daughter began menstruating we decided to celebrate this rite of passage by going out for an elegant dinner. We invited a friend of hers along, and the three of us ate Japanese food, chatted about their aspirations, plans and education, and talked about boys! We also played with a crystal pendulum, sharing a feminine oracular tradition.

MOON, A TRAVELLING woman in her 50's

When my oldest daughter started Bleeding, I don't remember any particular celebration. I was more inspired with my next daughter. When she started Bleeding, she was living with a friend close by and called to tell me she was Bleeding. The next time I saw her was in a busy setting at a country fair. I knew she was embarrassed by my being a witch and thought I was weird, and yet liked me and would always come to me for healing. So I went to see her and took her a big red rose, she asked me what it was for. I told her it was to celebrate her Bloods, and she said "Shhh! Not so loud!" There was no one around that could have heard; I didn't say it that loud. I was being considerate. She said, "What is the rose for?" and I said, "For your new pal." She said, "You mean my new problem."

Y.M., EXOTIC DANCER in her 30's; San Diego, CA

About ten years ago when I was living in California I belonged to a pagan women's circle. In that circle were a few women who had pretty traumatic first Blood experiences so we decided to do a healing ritual for all of us. After this long a time, some of the details of that ritual are pretty vague, but one thing that stands out for me were the dolls. We all made a little rag doll to represent ourselves as young girls. I still have mine; she sits on my dressing table and sometimes when I'm particularly upset, it's very comforting to hold her. I made my doll out of an old sheet and dressed her in a gown made from an old dress. I did this purposely so the cloth of the doll would have a lot of my vibes connected to it. I don't remember all the details of the ritual. I remember we had an archway which we (and our dolls) walked through to symbolize becoming a woman, and I remember sitting in the centre of the circle and each of us taking turns to tell our little girl doll-selves the facts about menstruation in the way we wished our mothers had told us. Unfortunately, that's all I remember about the ritual, except later we broke out some wine and had a really noisy good time. It was quite a meaningful experience that helped clear out a lot of old hassles for me and, I think, the others too. I'm sorry I can't remember any more but maybe this idea will inspire other women to create their own rituals in the same way.

❦

THE MOON CIRCLE WOMEN; Victoria, BC

R. was eleven when she and her father lived with me. She was the kind of girl who was so receptive that she was very open to us doing a ritual for her. I always had this fantasy about having a ritual for young girls. I believe puberty is a very important stage in a girl's life that should be celebrated. So when she started showing signs, budding breasts and hormones taking a flip, I asked her if she would like to celebrate her coming womanhood. She was delighted which was wonderful and not a typical reaction. We asked her what she wanted, but I think she just wanted us to do something for her. So, my women's group sat down with our ideas and some books to read and planned it. It started like this:

We've come tonight to celebrate womanhood, to strengthen and deepen the significance of the bodily and psychic changes that come with puberty. Tonight we celebrate with R. her passage into physical maturation and, with it, a new identification with the world of women. Many of us come here with a need to heal ourselves, for our own passages were times of confusion and fear, without support and understanding. We offer to R. our collective support for her transition, with our songs, our dance and our love.

What we did first was open the circle and welcome the Goddess and spirit guides of the four directions. Then we made a dedication, or statement of intent, regarding what we were there to do. We all wore white, which was very difficult to find in most of our closets. In the circle we had pink and white objects to symbolize the child. We chanted as we prepared R. We painted her face and someone had made her a garland of flowers with ribbons. She had on a beautiful white dress (actually my wedding dress). Then we invited her to dance the dance of the child to acknowledge that part of her. There was drumming as we stood all around her. Then our circle of women divided into two and we formed an arch. As R. began to pass through the arch, the women behind her broke apart and came forward to form a new circle in front of her. There was a real flow and feeling of support so as she moved into the adult circle there was always someone there to greet her.

This new circle we created was all red; red candles, red flowers and red foods (cherries, pomegranates and a wonderful, red, juice drink). When she entered into the women's circle, we all danced with her. There was also time for each woman to dance alone in the circle to celebrate her own coming of age.

At this point in the ritual we moved into an improvised chanting period. At one point we were just hooting and everybody felt really good. When we were all finished dancing and chanting, we sat down and gave her gifts. She was given a candle to light when she started Bleeding, a basket with pads in it, and a pretty necklace. At this time we shared with R. our own stories. We had talked about our transition periods before. For many women there was a real sense of pain surrounding this event in our lives. There had been no acknowledgement of the change.

We also did a tarot reading for her. Then we closed the circle. It was a real gift that R. had given us. I felt very proud of the whole experience.

⁊⁊⁊

S.B., ACUPUNCTURIST in her late 40's; Victoria, BC

The women's circle I go to periodically has a very simple, positive approach to first Blood. What they do, as each daughter comes of age, is make her a quilt. We each had squares that we embroidered, then the quilt was made and given to the young girl from the women's circle. At that time she was also invited to join us when her periods had started. It was like honouring her for becoming a woman and I thought that was just wonderful. This is a little different than focusing on the menstrual part. The focus was more on becoming a woman and being included in women's things. The young girls who did come to our women's circle loved it.

H.C., PSYCHOLOGIST in her 30's; Los Angeles, CA

I have recently read about newly reclaimed initiation rituals rooted in the Jewish tradition in a wonderful book called *Miriam's Well: Rituals for Jewish Women Around the Year* (by Penina Adelman, Biblio Press, 1986). Through this I learned that the idea of a girl's coming of age into womanhood is embodied in the Hebrew language, and, hence, in the ancient ways. A girl coming-of-age is called a "bogeret" and the coming-of-age is called a "bagrut." This is different from a "bar mitzvah," a more commonly known coming-of-age rite for boys. A bar mitzvah is initiation into the circle of the adult Jewish community, while a bogeret is specifically initiated into the circle of the community of women. The bagrut occurs shortly after a young woman's first Blood occurs.

The example given in this book suggests that a core aspect of the rite is the young woman giving a teaching to the older women. Specifically, she gives a teaching about the deeper, hidden meanings, symbolism, and roots of her Hebrew (ceremonial) name. This teaching (called a midrash) could be in the form of a talk, dance, song, poem, drama, or whatever the young girl is most comfortable with. The decision regarding how much she prepares and presents the teaching on her own, with the active support or input of her mother, can be decided individually, according to the maturity and comfort level of the initiate. Of course, it would also be very important that the rite include a time for the older women to share their stories and offer their blessings and gifts to the initiate as well.

What I liked about this idea is that, in teaching about the hidden meanings of her name, the initiate is taking an active part in her joining the circle of women. She contributes to the circle right from the start and thus truly moves into a new role and relatedness with these women. Also, by focusing on her own name for this teaching, the initiate is in a sense claiming herself. Her teaching (or midrash) about the deeper meaning of her name is a way of saying this is who I am. Certainly the process of preparation for such a teaching, and the presentation, would effectively focus the young woman and her mother on the true nature and meaning of the deeper levels of womanhood. And last, in the focus on hidden, deeper meanings of her name, the initiate and her circle are entering the realm of mystery, dream, symbol, revelation – all traditional provinces of Woman Wisdom.

◦◦◦◦◦

M.P.,TEACHER IN HER 40's; Nanaimo, BC

When my girls first had their periods, I gave them a sage bath. Then we sat down together and had a prayer circle. We smudged with sweet grass, prayed, and talked. At the closing of our circle I gave them each an eagle feather. I wanted to make this time special for them. In the old days there would have been a ceremony, but nowadays our people don't do anything to honour this event. I wanted to honour my girls' emerging adulthood. I wanted to give them the love and self-confidence I never had.

◦◦◦◦◦

K.J., NURSE AND MIDWIFE in her 40's; Portland, OR

I was drawn to tell you the story of my daughter's first Bloods. My own first Bleeding was one of shame and embarrassment. I didn't want to go to school or see anyone. I still remember seeing my underpants soaking in the bathtub, and I remember feeling ashamed. I didn't want anyone to know I was Bleeding.

I wanted my daughter's Bleeding to be special, not like mine. When she began to develop breasts and have pubic hair, I knew her time would come soon, so I started talking to her about Bleeding and what it meant to become a woman. I am a Lesbian and participate in women's circles so I knew we could do something special for her.

What I envisioned for her was a kind of magical transformation that would honour her emerging womanhood. Though I knew she was totally open to it the year before, two months before her periods actually began, she told me she didn't want to circle with my friends. Over that year I had been collecting a lot of gifts and red things for the ceremony but, when she told me how she felt, I knew that I had to put aside my own needs for a first Blood ritual, and honour who she was.

When she actually started Bleeding, it was really sad for me because I was away for that weekend. She told me later that she had noticed Blood on the towel when she showered so she just put on a pad and carried on with her life. It was five days before she told me this and she was afraid and embarrassed for having waited so long. A friend was with her when she told me. At first I didn't know what she was talking about. When I finally understood, I burst into tears. I was so excited and happy for her. I asked her when she started and was just devastated when she told me. I felt like I had failed her in some way because I hadn't been there to create that special time for her. I felt like a horrible mother. So, we held each other and cried and talked about how I hadn't been there for her and how she needed to take responsibility for her contributing to that situation. It was a lot of growing work for the both of us.

Then we talked about doing a ritual for her at the next new moon; not a large public ritual, just the two of us and a friend who was very special to her. The day came about ten days after her Bloods. The three of us went upstairs to my room where I have my altar. Even though I had collected all this stuff, the ritual itself was very spontaneous.

We began by holding hands and I presented my daughter to the Goddess. I sang a song and asked that she be received by the Goddess and that she be welcome as a woman. I felt so differently towards her. My heart felt so open to her, this young woman who was also my baby, my last child. It was such an opening of feeling, so exciting. We held hands, rocked and swayed and held our bellies. I had some of her first Blood on the altar which we cried over. We did a lot of crying; there was so much emotion. During the ritual I gave her her first medicine bag to fill with special rocks and other special medicines. Because my daughter's friend had such a negative time at her first period I presented her to the Goddess as well. This really bonded the friendship of these two young women who were taking this journey together, entering the circle of womanhood that includes all the women throughout time who have ever Bled.

Then we had red cake and cranberry juice and she opened the red packages and we draped her in red cloth. We laughed a lot and had fun. Afterwards we gathered once more around the altar to close the circle.

At present, my daughter's attitude towards her Blood isn't very spiritual, even though she honoured it during the ritual. It isn't an inconvenience – it just happens each month. She doesn't have pain; it doesn't get in her way.

RITUALS FOR CHILDREN, Cornwoman

This is actually the story of two rituals; the first giving rise to the second which was an actual first Blood ritual.

Last summer my six-year-old son's birthday fell on a full moon. Jes has always been the kind of kid who likes ritual and so I thought up the idea of giving him a moon party" in addition to the cake and ice cream he would have with his friends.

The moon party took place in the evening about nine o'clock. It was late, but in the summer moonrise and darkness come late here. Several of my friends gathered at my house. We picked up the ritual gear and headed down to a secluded beach about a mile from my home. As we walked, we sang songs and talked with Jes about his birthday. He was very excited because earlier that day, when we were baking cookies for the moon party, I told him that the Moon Goddess might come down from the sky to see him on his birthday.

When we got to the beach we laid out the four altars (North, South, East and West) complete with candles. A central altar with a Goddess statue, goblet of apple juice, and the moon cookies was also set up. Then, as priestess, I took Jes down to the water. He waded in with me, in his bathing suit, and I symbolically cleansed him by dipping a cedar bough in the ocean and sprinkling water over him. After Jes, everyone else was blessed in the same way. Then we dressed Jes in a white robe with a silver sash and placed a dark blue cape on his shoulders. I painted his face with a white crescent moon. We were now ready to begin. We cast the circle by honouring the four guardians of the directions. When we were inside the circle the moon began to rise over the ocean and we began to sing:

Goddess Moon, Holy Moon
come down to earth tonight.
Let me feel your fire
let me bathe in your light.

After we sang this for a while, a figure veiled in black and silver approached our circle. It was the Moon Goddess (actually a dear friend of mine who had been briefed ahead of time). Slowly She approached the circle.

She asked if a boy named Jesse was among us. I brought him forward to kneel before Her. I told Her he was my son and that I dedicated him to Her. I said other things on the spur of the moment which I can't remember now.

It was very meaningful to me because, like Jes, I imagined not my friend, but the actual Goddess there before us. The Lady asked if Jes could walk with Her along the beach. I opened the circle and he went with Her. What they talked about on that magical stroll is Jes' s secret. When he returned he showed us that She had given him several little gifts, including a moonstone placed in a beautiful, crocheted bag. We said goodbye to the Goddess and I closed the circle again, once Jes was back inside. After that, Jes passed around the cookies and apple juice. We talked and others gave him gifts as well. The moon was much higher now. It was a wonderful night. The reflection on the water was marvelous. The adults could have stayed up for hours longer, talking and watching the moon, but it was late and Jes was tired and restless, so we opened the circle and went home. Weeks later, he still was talking about the visit from the Moon Goddess. Some of our non-pagan friends thought he was a bit weird, so I told him to keep it a secret, just for us to know. All in all, it was a very special night that he will always remember.

I describe this ritual in such detail to make a couple of points, the first being that you can do, and should do, ritual with young children. The second is that doing rituals, like the moon party, earlier in life will get a young girl used to the idea of doing a ritual when her first Blood comes.

Later that summer, a woman who was at Jes's party asked me to help her create a ritual for her daughter who had just started her period. This is what we did.

Prior to the first Blood ritual, Lisa and her mom prepared little gifts to give to the participants in the ceremony. It is a Native Indian custom to give out gifts as part of religious events. Behind this custom is the thought that, if a person asks for something in the ceremony, the gift will have more meaning for that person if she has focused healing energies ahead of time by preparing gifts for the participants in the ritual. In this case, the gifts were moon cookies (cookies in the shapes of full and crescent moons), and little red pouches filled with cornmeal.

With the help of some friends, Lisa's mother made her a ritual dress. There was a lot of time spent talking about the rite while sewing it, and we asked for Lisa's opinion so she would feel she'd contributed to its creation. When the day finally arrived, we were all ready. The moon was in the wrong phase to do a night ritual, so we chose to do the ceremony at dawn. At about four o'clock, we gathered and walked down to the same beach of Jes's moon party. There was no one about that early in the morning. We set up our circle in the Wiccan way, then went down to bathe in the sea.

As the sun rose, we held hands and walked into the ocean singing. It was very beautiful, but also very cold, so we took a quick dip, then rushed out laughing. We dressed Lisa in her ritual dress with a red sash at her waist. We braided ribbons in her hair and painted her face with red paint and a white crescent moon. As we dressed her we sang to her but there was no chit chat. All our energy was focused on creating the ritual space. I've seen gossipy talk drain away the power of a ritual too many times, and we wanted everything to be just right for our young maiden. When she was dressed, her mother blindfolded her and bound her wrists and led her out of sight down the beach. [This part of the ritual conforms to the initiation ordeal stage of the shamanic transformation process. Confronting fear is a necessary element in all rites of passage and, if an initiation rite does not contain this element, the sense of a threshold experience is not attained and a successful transition is unlikely.] Lisa was placed on a rock near the shore. Blindfolded and bound, she was to wait there for the Goddess (Dark Moon Woman) to come and release her and return her to the women's circle. As she sat, her mother told her to think about her childhood that was passing away and her womanhood that was approaching. She was to remain where she was until the Goddess came for her. Then she left Lisa and returned to the circle.

After Lisa's mother returned, we gathered in the sacred circle. We did a breathing meditation and smudged ourselves with sage and mugwort. We called in the four guardians and invoked the blessing of the Goddess. We drummed and danced and sang, raising energy and giving Lisa time to experience her blindfolded condition up the beach. No one kept track of time, but Lisa probably stayed out there at least an hour before, masked and ritually robed, the figure of the Goddess went up the beach to fetch her.

As Lisa sat blindfolded and bound, Dark Moon Woman, the Goddess of the Blood, came and touched her. She removed the girl's bonds (but not her blindfold) saying:

In your childhood you were bound by the love and disciplines of your family. As you become a woman, you must be responsible for the discipline of your own body and be bound by the love of all life. You must always treat yourself with love and respect. Within your womb lies the gift of creation and the blessed Blood of life.

Dark Moon Woman led Lisa back to the waiting circle of women, and told her that, when we come into this world as women, we are given the gift of creation like the Earth, Herself, but we also have the responsibility to take care of the Earth and the beings that live on the Earth. As women, we do this by remaining grounded to the Earth, open to hearing the voice of the Earth speak to us through our Bleeding each month. When a woman Bleeds, she should be quiet and rest, allowing the Earth mother to communicate with her, either through her dreams or in meditation. As they neared the circle, Dark Moon Woman reached down and picked up a flat rock about the size of her palm. She gave it to Lisa and told her to keep it and each month she could place it on her belly. She should breathe deeply so that she could feel the rock move up and down. This would help her always to be in touch with her womb and the Goddess within her.

Dark Moon Woman led Lisa to the circle and removed her blindfold saying:

As a child you were blinded by your innocence. As a young woman you must see to make your own choices in life. As a child you have come here. As a woman, go forth now.

When Lisa opened her eyes she saw the women lined up in an arch (or birth canal) to welcome her into the women's circle. The Goddess led her to the birth canal and then said goodbye. As Lisa passed through, the women whispered blessings and hugged and kissed her, welcoming her into the circle as a woman. As she passed into the circle, her mother greeted her with a hug, then gave Lisa a beautiful pendant containing a moonstone and a carnelian set in silver. She also held out a bowl in which menstrual Blood had been mixed with cornmeal. She marked her daughter's forehead with the Blood explaining that by this bond of Blood, all women are united, and that by this Blood, is the wisdom of the ages passed on to the next generation.

The drum had been beating softly during all this like an ancient echoing voice to our words. Now it burst forth again in a loud, lively rhythm. We began to sing and dance. We encouraged Lisa to dance for us. It was very beautiful! As the sun grew higher and we wilted in the heat, we sat and passed around the offering cup of ritual Blood red juice (strawberry in this case). As each woman drank she told Lisa briefly how it had been for her at her first Blood. It was a very moving time for all of us.

When we finished, Lisa thanked us and gave to each of us her gifts of the red pouches and cookies. These gifts symbolized the love, creativity and power she would bring to us with the gift of her Moon Blood each month. After this we closed the circle and went back to Lisa's house where Lisa's dad and younger brother had prepared a meal of red foods for us. It was a wonderful day for all. It felt so good to change the pattern of fear and ignorance which most of us experienced at our first Blood.

As a postscript I might add, that if an older woman had a very traumatic first Blood experience, she could exorcise much of those old feelings by having a similar ritual done for her. As you begin the ritual, do a guided (trance) visualization to put her back in time so that she can act out the experience in the way she wishes it could have been. Through the medium of the ritual, recreate the past as it should have been.

THE RITE OF PASSAGE into Womanhood,
De-Anna Alba

In preparing your daughter for the ritual it will be necessary for her to take a ritual bath. It would be a good idea if you also took one. Draw a tub of warm water and put in a few drops of musk oil. This represents an earthy scent associated with the Earth mother and your daughter's growing sexuality. An alternative you can add is rosemary water or rosemary herb itself to symbolize the Goddess and the home. Float red and white flowers in the water. The red represents the flow of her cycles, the white represents the purity and beauty of this welcome and natural process.

Burn some incense in the room. The choice of scent is yours, although Frankincense is recommended since it is a well known purifier of the mind, body and spirit. Since she will be brought into the presence of the Lady, it is important that she be purified with the incense as well as the water.

Burn three candles – two red and one white (the colour symbolism is the same as for the flowers). Three is a sacred number to the Goddess and it also represents the phases of the moon, an integral part of our monthly cycles.

Lay out some red and white clothing for her to wear. When she goes in to take a bath you say something like:

Today is a very special day for you. We celebrate the birth of your womanhood for you have recently begun your monthly cycles of Bleeding.

Tell her about the symbolism of all the trappings in the room including the water itself which represents the great womb of the Goddess in which we are all safely kept. Tell her about these things as she relaxes in the water.

Once she is dressed, take her into a room lit only by candle-light, with flowers and incense burning on a table draped in a white cloth. You will also need a chalice of some sort on the table, filled with either menstrual Blood or dark red wine.

At the North point of the room place an unlit green candle far enough from the wall for you to stand behind and a green ribbon or green yam about 1-1/2 feet long. Do the same for each of the other directions: a yellow candle and ribbon in the East; a red candle and ribbon in the South; and a blue candle and ribbon in the West. In the middle, place an unlit white candle, white ribbon, pair of scissors or knife, and a gift. Have two additional lit, white candles on the table. Play appropriate music softly in the background (Kay Gardner's Moon Circles or Georgia Kelly's Sea Peace album are both good).

Go into the room with your daughter and stand or sit in front of the white draped table. Say the following:

This is a special time in your life and marks your passage into the fellowship of all women. Not only have you become part of womankind, but you have become as one with the Great Goddess, the Divine Mother. You are beginning to go through bodily changes on a monthly cycle only to begin growing again. You ebb and flow like the sea, a symbol of our Goddess/Mother. As you look up to the sky and see the ever-changing phases of the Moon, you are reminded nightly of the flux of your body and Hers.

You are now a woman grown and able to bring forth life from your body, just as the Goddess brought forth the plants, animals, and the first people of this

Earth, even giving birth to the Earth itself. You are a daughter of the Divine Mother and a vessel of creation, and as such, are thrice Blessed.

At this point, anoint her third eye with the menstrual Blood or wine from the chalice and say:

First, as your Blood has begun to flow, so now will your intuition and psychic ability grow.

Now anoint her heart with the Blood and say:

Second, now that your body has proclaimed its maturity, so too will your heart begin to be filled with a nurturing kindness and love that only a woman can give.

Now anoint the solar plexus, the region of the stomach or womb, with the Blood and say:

Third, because your body is now fertile, the gift of life is yours to give. Use it wisely, as this gift can be given in your care before you are ready to accept it graciously and before you are ready to care for it like the priceless treasure it is.

Take her by the hand and say:

Now is the time for you to meet our Divine Mother in some of Her many guises.

Lead her to the yellow candle in the East. Have her stand in front of it and you behind it. Tell her that, as part of womankind, you are an earthly living representative of the Goddess, and as such will be the voice of the Goddess and speak for Her. (In other words, She will speak through you-you become a medium for Her message.)

Have your daughter light the yellow candle, and then you, as the Goddess, say something like:

I am the laughing Goddess of the wind and have come this day to celebrate the day of your birth and the day of your rebirth as a young woman, and since it is your birthday, I have brought you the gift of wisdom that you may judge properly all you see, feel and hear.

Tie the yellow ribbon around her wrist leaving a long tail hanging down. Hug her, kiss her, take her by the hand, and move to the South. Have her light the red candle and say something like:

I am the warm and shining Goddess of the Sun and I bring you the gift of love that you may spend your days surrounded by those whom you love and those who love you.

Tie the red ribbon around her wrist, leaving a tail hanging down. Hug her, kiss her, take her by the hand, and go to the West. Have her light the blue candle and say the following:

I am the Star of the Sea and Goddess of the laughing waters. I bring you the gift of intuition that you may understand the problems of others and of yourself and thus be better able to solve them.

Tie the blue ribbon on with the others, again leaving a long tail. Hug her, kiss her, take her by the hand, and walk to the North. Have her light the green candle and listen to the words:

I am the mighty Earth Mother and creatrix of all. I bring you the gift of life and growth that you may continue to grow and unfold the wonders that you are, and that, one day, you may give life to another just as your mother has done for you and her mother before her, all the way back to the beginnings of Woman on Earth.

Tie the green ribbon around her wrist, again leaving a tail. Hug her, kiss her, take her by the hand, and go to the centre. Have her light the white candle and say something like this:

I am the Great Goddess, the Divine Mother of all that is, was, and ever shall be. I bring you the gift of spiritual purity, the knowledge that you are my divine daughter and as such, are greatly loved by me. Know also that there is a deep inner part of you that is a part of me and will be in constant touch with me for the rest of your life and for many lifetimes to come.

Tie the white ribbon around her wrist and say something like:

This spiritual essence is that which binds each part of you to yourself and to all Womankind, just as it binds all these Goddess-given gifts together as a whole.

Braid all the ribbons together leaving enough room to tie a knot at the bottom of the braiding and still leave about five inches of the tail. Then say a prayer to the Goddess yourself, commending your daughter to Her loving care. Use any words you feel appropriate or use the following:

Gracious Goddess, Divine Mother of us all, hold my daughter close to your heart. Teach her the mysteries of life. Make her proud of her sex and her Woman heritage. Help her to understand that her Bleeding is a natural and wonderful part of her nature and to never be ashamed of it, but to be proud and happy in the knowledge that this wondrous gift of life has been placed into her safekeeping.

At the end of the prayer, pour a little of the wine or Blood from the chalice into the incense burner as an offering to the Goddess.

Be seated again by the white candle and give her your gift. This should be something red that she can wear every time she has her Moon. For example, a special ring set with a red stone such as garnet or even a red piece of glass or synthetic red stone. It should look nice, as she will probably wear it during her Moon for the rest of her life.

⟨❦⟩

BLENDING MANY CULTURES in a Gift of Love,
Rachel Wallace

At the four crossroads, ten women of the Svaha Lodge gather under a starry sky. We stand in ceremonial dress, each uniquely adorned in symbols of our own personal journey on the spiral dance of life. We have prepared ourselves for this female rite of passage, and we wait, alert and expectant. The signal will come from Judy, whose seventeen-year-old Scandinavian exchange student, Mette, has asked us for an initiation, a rite of passage, into womanhood.

Ceremonies are not new to us – we've incorporated ritual into our women's group to celebrate collective and personal transitions and transformations. But this one is special – I can see it in my sisters' faces. This is a rite of passage not only for our collective daughter, but also for ourselves and, in some unexplained way, for the women of the world. It is the initiation we yearn for in a time that is past; it is the healing for the deep, collective wound that cries for balm.

The drumming starts softly, a muffled heartbeat of the universe, and we begin a chant that one of us has written for this rite:

We bring our daughter
We bring our daughter
Our woman way
Our woman way

Slowly, we begin walking down the rural road towards Judy's home, imagining that the drumming and chanting is subtly slipping into Mette's unconscious before she is alerted to our presence. Soon, we are at the door;

Judy, as Mette's symbolic mother, and Judith and Linda, her handmaidens for the evening, enter. Chanting, they move towards her room. She is sitting on the bed, and her blue eyes are wide; she has known only that the ceremony would take place within these last two days. Her eyes tell the three women that she now wonders what she has gotten herself into. But she is brave, this woman from a far off place. Judy asks, "Mette, are you ready to embrace your womanhood?" Mette answers, "Yes." The ceremonial blanket is wrapped around her shoulders, red diamonds on grey wool representing the red of menses, the red of Mother's Blood, the red of passion. Linda and Judith lead her from the room.

We climb into our van to travel the mile to the Lodge, a snug circle with Mette in the middle, and chant our way down the road. Once there, leaving the outer world behind, we take off our shoes and enter this special, sacred place that has held us and nurtured us so gently over the last few years. Tonight, the room is filled with the scent of our Earth's sacred herbs, of burning sage and cedar. As we move into our customary circle, we breathe in the beauty of the room and each other and smile.

Judy steps to the centre of the circle to open the ceremony with a blessing, a statement of our sacred intent. Though we often interweave masculine and feminine energies, tonight she calls upon the female powers of the four directions, and of the sky, the earth and the moon. She lights sage inside a large sea shell. It flames, then smoulders as she blows out the flame. The smoke, the breath of the Great Spirit, the breath of Life, rises as if it is indeed a spirit. Slowly, Judy walks around the circle with the shell of sage and a large feather, smudging each woman. [Smudging refers to the practice of waving sage or sweetgrass smoke over someone, in order to cleanse and purify their spirit.] Sage of the earth, bird of the air, embers of the fire, shell of the water, the elements join us. Some of us simply breathe the smoke; others gently fan it over our bodies in this ancient ritual of purification. We feel ourselves begin to move to a deeper level of reality.

Tonight's rituals have been chosen with Mette in mind. We have created some specifically for her; others evolved from our experience. We've done the intellectual work by preparing the evening in detail, always focusing on making it a positive, but challenging, experience for this young woman we are beginning to know and love. I wonder how she will receive these goings-on. Might we unintentionally offend her? Frighten her? Judy has prepared her as best she could by sharing with her some of the things we do, but now it is time to let go and simply do it with as great a love as we can find.

We sit on the floor and begin a series of culturally and religiously diverse chants and songs as we continue our deepening, accompanying ourselves with drums, rattles, bells, and tambourines. We sing each chant for several minutes, aiming for that seven-minute length when the brain's neo-cortex lets go and primal connections begin. I become aware of voices deepening and gaining power as the ancient parts of ourselves begin to stir. Now the sound comes from the solar plexus, the belly, not the throat. We are singing with our souls; we are singing women of Mother Earth; we are singing women of power and strength.

When the chanting subsides, Judy asks Mette the initiatory questions: As a woman, what do you wish to receive from this world? As a woman, what will you contribute to it? She has prepared an answer which she speaks from her heart, and it touches us deeply. We respond with "amen", "ho", "blessed be", and "may it always be so." Linda asks Mette for her giveaway and she teaches us a lullaby in Danish. [The "giveaway" is the gift one brings to the spirit of the ritual, a gesture of gratitude and respect.] Suddenly, I am struck by the paradox: we are birthing this woman, birthing her from childhood into womanhood, and she has provided the birthing song.

Linda's voice brings me back to the ceremony. We wish Mette to enter womanhood with dreams, she says. What are our dreams for her? She invites Mette to the centre of our circle and we make ourselves comfortable around her. Linda uses her gift of storytelling to guide us on a meditative journey. Once at our inner destination, we let images rise from the unconscious to tell us of our dreams for Mette. When we finish, we do not speak, but chant quietly as Carol and Sue leave to prepare the sweatlodge.

Ten minutes later we walk down a winding path partly lit with candles, down the hill, through the firs, our bare feet on the damp, cool earth.

The blazing fire, that heats the rocks, crackles and dances outside the sweatlodge. The candle-lit outbuilding is cold, and we shiver in silence as we fold our clothes and wrap ourselves in towels. Mette's handmaidens take her clothes and fold them gently, laying them carefully in a basket. They wrap the ceremonial blanket around her as if they were mothers tenderly swaddling their child. We walk to the sweatlodge with Mette nestled in the middle of the line. The grass is cold and wet; the fire illuminates the blankets covering the low dome of the sweatlodge.

We gather in front of the East-facing entrance, where I explain the practical aspects of the lodge as minimally as I can. Then I say:

Prepare yourselves to enter this most female of holy places: the womb of Mother Earth. Here, we invoke the spirits, and the spirits come. Here, we cleanse ourselves, we die and are reborn. Here, we pray, we sing, we stretch ourselves to endure the heat, dark, and steam. Here, we offer our support and our dreams for Mette, and in doing so, we remember, we re-vision our own entry into womanhood.

Sue steps forward to offer water to the four directions, the sky and the Earth, pouring some upon the Earth, asking that it purify us in this special sweat. She raises it to the new moon, the perfect symbol of new womanhood, in homage.

We enter the low door on our knees, moving counter-clockwise, the direction of the feminine in many cultures. The dim, earthy lodge is already hot from the pile of glowing rocks that the firetenders, Carol and Sue, have placed in the centre hole, the navel of the Great Mother. Mette enters last, her handmaidens at each side. She sits by the door, the coolest place, though hot by any standard once the steam begins. Linda lets down the door canvas and blanket; suddenly all traces of reflected firelight are gone. The rocks no longer glow, and it is incredibly dark in this womb of our rebirth. We are about to take another step into the primal depths. We are about to return to our source, the Great Mother, Mother Earth.

I check with Mette, then everyone else, to see how they're doing. Mette sounds good; I realize her experience with Scandinavian saunas has been helpful. There is a transitional silence and I begin the sweat with a prayer.

Carol pours water across the rocks; they sizzle and hiss as an unseen cloud of steam rises and moves outward toward us, blasting us with a wall of heat. We begin easy, but, even so, the heat takes our breath. There are groans as we adjust. I find my voice and begin the Sumash Indian chant which calls the spirits to the sweatlodge, feeling the sound vibrate through me and around me as others join in. I signal the end of the eight rounds with my rattle and begin the Chant of White Buffalo Woman, the female aspect of the Great Spirit in Sioux tradition. After the opening chants, the women periodically offer songs from their own spiritual journeys. These are gifts to the Great Spirit in gratitude for blessings seen and unseen, known and unknown. These are gifts for Mette, too, given from our hearts and souls.

More water dances unseen on the rocks. As the heat grows, the sweat begins to pour off our bodies. We pass around water to drink, offering it with care and love to the woman next to us. Mette indicates that she's okay; one of our sisters who has difficulty with the heat scrunches down to the ground to breathe cooler air. Although we know we can leave at any time, we all intend to stay. A few of us have been in excruciatingly hot sweats and we know that the visions often come after the point at which we think we can no longer bear the heat and steam. But the intention tonight is to challenge ourselves gently.

"What are our dreams for Mette?" I ask as the water comes full circle. We begin to share, one by one, describing the images that came to us. The dreams are rich, beautiful, touching, and sometimes funny. These are woman images, thick with meaning for us. Some of us cry at their poignancy, for they come from our souls and they speak of what we want for ourselves as well. We sing a favourite song, one which speaks of our hopes and dreams for ourselves, for Mette, and for each other.

As more water hisses on the rocks, I open the sweat to spontaneous prayers. They come from all around the circle; prayers coming from women's open hearts. "Mother /Father God, may this be so for Mette," "Wakantanka, may this be so for us," and "Jesus, hear our prayers." The intimacy of shared dreams speaks in our prayers. "Heart's desire, Thy Will be done."

Somewhere in that inner place of knowing, we intuitively sense that Mette, the child, has moved into womanhood. Starting quietly, then building, we chant:

Strong woman, wise woman
Earth woman, sky woman

A final pouring of water on our sacred rocks and we begin the last round of the sweat. "We welcome you to womanhood, Mette, I say, now that you are a woman, you are our sister, and we offer you our stories." We begin to share our wisdom from our womanhood, and how we learned it – wisdom from pain, wisdom from joy. "Wise woman, woman wise, embers burning in ancient eyes." We sing Mette's lullaby, now our lullaby, as we draw the birthing sweat to a close, finishing with a group prayer of gratitude.

"Sisters, we are being birthed into the world as new women," I say. "Let us leave the womb." We crawl out on our knees and try to stand on the wobbly legs of newborns. We reach for jugs of ice cold water to wash the sweat away. The icy water is a shock, like a first breath in a new world. I fall to the ground, arms outstretched, to embrace the belly of Mother Earth. Later, we stand around the outdoor fire that burns like the fire inside us now. To the Great Spirit, we give deep and enduring thanks.

When the time is right, we return to the outbuilding to dress; Judith and Linda offer Mette beautiful new silk undergarments, then wrap her again in the ceremonial blanket. We walk up the hill to Svaha Lodge, where we dress her in her ceremonial costume, a gift to her from the women. She is adorned with symbols of life, symbols of womanhood, jewelry of feathers, beads, and shells. We laugh, sing, and talk, filled with joy at her joy, her beauty, her big, wide open grin. Dee has brought food and drink; we begin singing and telling our stories.

We end the evening with a circle, arm in arm. I wonder how much time has passed; it feels like days, like years, like lifetimes, like minutes. The mysterious healing power of the ceremony strikes me to the heart as tears flow down our faces. We have midwifed not only Mette, but ourselves and Everywoman.

Our daughter is a woman now, and our lives are different because of it. Mette has gone through the rite of passage – the rite we never had, never held in our memory, but now do.

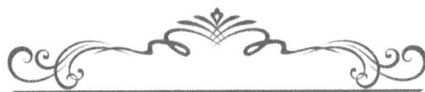

The Bloods

Power Gift

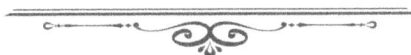

THERE IS POWER IN THE Blood of all woman
There is power in the Blood that transforms us
There is joy in the gift of our Blood

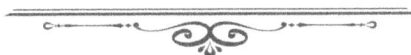

I WAS IN CALIFORNIA a few years ago, attending a workshop with Starhawk, when I discovered my Bloods as a time of power. On the final night of the program, all the women in my group planned to have a concluding ritual. We decided to use a Blood anointing as part of our rite. It was interesting to note that by the end of our week together, seven of the thirteen women in our group were Bleeding, no matter when our periods might have been normally scheduled to come. I came ten days ahead of my normal cycle, so I was one of the seven who saved Blood on the last day to contribute to the ritual. Coming from a Native background, where menstruation means total isolation from sacred ceremonies, it was quite a shock. To actually use Moon Blood in a ritual was a totally revolutionary idea for me and I liked it. Being actually anointed by the Blood was also very meaningful for me. I felt transformed. It was like receiving confirmation of something I had known inside all my life. A great weight of fear and guilt was lifted from my shoulders, and I knew I needed to explore this further when I returned home.

After this ritual, many changes started happening in my life as I pursued information on this subject. What I found out early in my quest was that there was not a lot of literature written that dealt with menstruation in a positive way. I realized that if I was to learn anything meaningful, the information would have to come from within.

The first thing I began doing was paying attention to my body rhythms. I charted when my period came, how I felt, and any important dreams or events that happened. Later, I charted the entire month rather than just my Bloods. In this way, I could see the larger perspective of my whole cycle. I had always been very lucky, I thought. My periods were as regular as a clock and they never hurt. I basically ignored them and thought I was very liberated by my attitude. What I realized, after doing my charts and meditations for a few months, was that there are two extreme reactions women can choose to have toward their periods. First, they can ignore them (as I chose to) and go on about business as usual, or they can have extremely painful periods that make it impossible to ignore them. Each of these conditions is an extreme in the swing of the pendulum. I now think each is equally undesirable. During a woman's period, she does change; that is an undeniable fact. Her emotional tolerance of stress, her energy levels, her creativity patterns, not to mention her body, all change like the ebb and flow of the tides. What I have learned to do is to work with my bodily tides rather than ignore or fight them as so many women do. In this way, I learned to make my cycle creative and empowering, rather than a curse.

As I worked with my cycle, a lot of healing and growth took place for me. During my Moon time, I began to know the figure of the Goddess within me, whom I called Dark Moon Woman. She began giving me Her songs and teachings which have, over the years, powerfully influenced my life. The one point that became so clear to me, and that I feel is one of the most important gifts of this book, is what Dark Moon Woman told me once, after a particularly humiliating isolation at a Native ceremony. She told me:

Your milk flows from your breasts when you have a child; you feed and nurture with this blessed liquid. Your Blood, too, is a nurturing liquid and if your family was starving, you could feed your children with your Blood as you did when you had milk. Your body wouldn't feed the fetus growing in your womb on poisons. This Blood that flows each month is not a way of getting rid of poisons from your body. It is a blessed liquid of nurturance.

In the times when a child isn't growing inside your womb, the Blood flows out as a sacred 'giveaway' that should be offered to care for other life on this

Earth. This Moon Blood is a sacred gift, not to be wasted or disposed of lightly. This sacred Blood should be returned to the Earth.

In exchange for this gift of Blood, a woman may receive spirit power and vision should she choose to seek it. Such gifts of the Blood should be used for the good of the people and will, in turn, be a blessing for all living things. This is the gift of the Moon Blood.

These words felt so right to me; I could feel it deep down in my belly. Since that time I have dedicated my life to sharing what I know with others.

J.Z.N., PSYCHIC READER in her 40's; Victoria, BC

I have to say I really like menstruating. Working with the psychic circle as I do I can't stop working just because I'm menstruating. I have found it an excellent time to do readings as I feel really sensitized. I get very rooted. I feel as though I turn into a tree when I'm doing readings while menstruating as I'm very solid and grounded. My readings are usually quite accurate as well.

I also have some very intense and prophetic dreams just prior to Bleeding. Some are warning dreams; others indicate the beginning of a new cycle and the cleansing of the old. It's also amazing that other people have had dreams for me just around my Bleeding time. I guess I also practice sex magic. I think it just naturally follows the whole tantric idea of sexuality as devotional practice.

One of the keys in magic is the intent and the emotion behind it. The movement of force outward from the body is the act of creating a circle. I feel that menstruating women really do give off an aura (a lot of energy) so I like to direct it sometimes. I've found that menstrual magic works best toward healing and issues pertaining to the body rather than for an affirmation of prosperity and light. My body makes a big deal out of menstruation. I've done some really long private rituals of seven hours just sitting in circle. I might do some oracular work and I do a lot of visualizations around resolving or exploring issues in my life. I also like to do astral travel and telepathic work. I like to work at night with the energy of the dark.

I have a little story about my athalme. I won't go into the whole story but, for years, I saw it in my dreams and in my mind's eye. Finally I found it, and it was absolutely perfect; just as I had imagined it. After I got it, I didn't consecrate it for a long time. I don't know why; I was waiting for the right time. Finally one night I was moved to do it, and I inscribed my knife with runes drawn with my menstrual Blood. Since that time, no one has picked up that knife. The Blood, of course, has dried up and gone away so no one knows it is there. People will pick up other things from my altar which aren't as meaningful, but interestingly enough, the knife hasn't been touched. There has to be something to that.

I like setting up an altar in my bathroom and taking a bath while Bleeding. I have a very heavy flow that really tinges the water. I find it very gratifying. I feel like I've participated in something really sacred.

I have this thing about Blood sacrifice and the sacrament of Blood. I feel that if we all were to realize that yes, in a sense, as a price for living in the physical expression on this planet, there will be Blood extracted. When we eat meat or plants, they have Blood as well; it's a different colour, but Blood nonetheless. When we eat, there is this very intimate giving back Blood to the Earth. I see other people have the same idea because I see those bumper stickers that say "War is menstruation envy." When we move beyond the need to be making war, when we get beyond killing each other, then menstruation will be recognized as that Blood that we at the end of the food chain give back to the Earth. I feel very strongly about that.

◎◈◈◎

K.J., NURSE AND MIDWIFE in her 40's; Portland, OR

When I fell in love with Amy, who lives on the land, I would go to be with her. I would see her squat or stand to pee. She would just spread her legs and squirt her urine. I was just blown away by how she could just open her pelvis and direct the flow of urine. She would also squat on the ground to Bleed. It was really eye opening to me because I was raised to keep my legs together and be a proper lady. So seeing this as part of her daily life was a really important lesson for me.

Because I'm involved with birthing, I know a woman will automatically open her legs when the baby is ready to come. That is the sign I look for. Some women, however, are so locked into keeping their legs closed that I literally have to pry their legs apart to receive the child. This is not unusual because we are so trained to keep our legs closed and not to show that part of ourselves.

❧

S., WITCH IN HER 50'S; San Francisco, CA

As a Wiccan, I have almost taken for granted that Moon time is a time of power and celebration. For us, it is when women are most in touch with energy flow and therefore it is a time when a woman would act as central priestess for a ritual. The idea behind this is that the woman's flow is the closest physical parallel to the natural cycle that exists. When a woman can produce Blood, she offers physical proof of the link with the Earth. Needless to say, only woman can do this, so their role is special.

The idea of cloistering or separating women from others during women's Moon time comes from a time when women chose to go away and celebrate this gift with other women, the mystery of it not being for men. Anne Cameron's book *Daughters of Copper Woman* contains stories of the creation of women in all societies and, specifically, women's power regarding Moon flow customs.

It is important to remember that when women did go away, it was not because they were sinful or unclean. Ironically, no ceremonies were held during that time because men were not in charge of spiritual life and could not perform the ceremonies without women.

❧

C.C., WITCH IN HER 30's; Oregon

Prohibitions about sex with a woman on her Moon are widespread and are linked to prohibitions about sex (from which a pregnancy can occur) at certain moon phases. I think the prohibitions were really to do with the instructions on how to get pregnant (or not) and were originally practical.

❧

C.E., TEACHER IN HER 40's; Northwest Territories

I married a Dene man from the Northwest Territories. One of the first things my mother-in-law and sister-in-law did when I stayed at their house was to instruct me on proper womanly behaviour. Among the Dene, there are certain things women shouldn't do. For example, a woman never crawls over her husband, she should go down to the foot of the bed and get out that way. When Dene women have their periods, they don't go off as they used to, but they shouldn't cook for men, or use the same face-cloth, towel, or washbasin as the rest of the family. I remember one time a woman came over to my mother-in-law's. I couldn't understand what they were talking about in their language but the woman was very angry. Later I asked my sister-in-law about it. She said the woman was angry because her daughter-in-law was acting like a white woman. She would wash herself in the same basin as the rest of the family while menstruating. Everyone in the house was sick because of it. She blamed the girl's unclean practices for all the family's trouble.

When I lived among the Native people, it seemed like menstruating women got blamed for a lot that went wrong in their communities. I never could take it too seriously, but I did try to observe the customs while I lived there.

⚬⚬⚬

L.G., NATIVE COURT worker in her 30's; Manitoba

Last summer I went to a Native ceremony out in the bush. There was an old grandmother there they called Turtle Woman. She talked to the women about spiritual things and, for the first time, I felt I understood why women weren't supposed to go to the sweatlodge, or other rituals, when they are in their Moon. Before, I had always been told these things by a man, or by a woman who got it all mixed up. I would always feel very confused or ashamed or angry. What Turtle Woman said was that when a woman Bleeds she is like a beacon. She is radiating energy while attracting energy at the same time. If the woman is in balance, she will give off the strong powers of love and peace-but if the woman is suffering from co-dependency, or drug and alcohol addiction, or is out of balance in some other way, she will broadcast sickness and unhappy feelings. If she goes near people during her

Moon, she will also be more likely to pick up things from them, too, if they are drinking or feeling bad.

This point was made clear to me when I went back to my job at the Native friendship centre because there is a girl who works there that showed me what Turtle Woman meant. I don't know this woman very well, but I can tell she has a lot of personal problems. Normally you can feel that, but when she is Bleeding it is much worse. I started to notice on those days that within a hour after she came to work, people around her would start having headaches or pick minor fights with each other. The woman herself wasn't bitchy or anything, she just was in a lot of physical and emotional pain at those times and other people would unconsciously pick it up and respond to her energy. I realized that menstruation is not the real problem, it is neither harmful nor harmless-it is merely a magnifier ten times over of what is inside the woman herself. I understand now why the old people have to be so careful – if that young woman from my work were to go to a sweat while in her Moon, and give off such energy, she could make someone sick without meaning to because in the sweat you are so open to everything.

I think we as women need to understand this and take more responsibility for our feelings during our Moon time. We need to honestly work on our own garbage and be aware that we may be influencing other people at this time.

⊖≪≫

MOON BLOOD FROM A NATIVE Perspective,
Cornwoman

I come from a mixed parentage of Native and European ancestry. Growing up as a Métis (half-breed) isn't easy for anyone, male or female, but as a woman, it seemed especially confusing. I received, and still do receive, a lot of mixed messages about being a woman from both sides of my family. Many white people I know have very romantic notions about Native philosophy and culture. Looking at my Native heritage realistically, I see both its good and bad points. As a Native, I learned good things from the Elders, including the necessity to respect and honour the Mother Earth and all life. Such teachings were very good, but the teachings I learned about being a woman have a darker and more confusing colour. I learned that as a woman my body was sacred because it brought forth life. I also learned that my woman's Blood, each month, was very powerful, but that it was also very dangerous and frightening. I was taught that if I wasn't careful I could make people around me sick just by my presence. When I was younger this was frightening to me because I could be accused of doing something that wasn't a deliberate or conscious act, but an unavoidable result of my Bleeding. How many times have I heard someone say, when a ceremony went wrong and someone got sick, "There must have been a menstruating woman there."

Though it varies from Nation to Nation, menstrual taboos are still very strong in traditional Native cultures. Today, when a woman is on her Moon time, she cannot participate in a religious ceremony such as the Pipe Ceremony, Big House Dance, Sun Dance, or Sweatlodge. She cannot touch a sacred object or prepare food which will be used in the ritual. The fear of menstrual Blood goes to unbelievable extremes with some Sioux medicine men who will keep their sacred objects in metal tool boxes in order to protect them from the power of a "Bleeding woman."

Growing up as a half-breed in an urban environment for much of my life, it has been difficult for me to understand this deep rooted fear which both Native men and women have of menstrual Blood. When I question people about their feelings on this issue, they get angry. They tell me it has always been that way and not to ask questions like a white woman. What can I say to that?

I have heard from some Elders that women don't need to go on a Vision Quest because each month their Bleeding cleanses their body, getting rid of all the poisons. Personally, I question that. I think this belief comes from a Christian idea that anything which comes out of the body between the legs is dirty and full of poisons. I don't accept that this is a pre-contact Native Indian belief but is one imposed on us by the invaders. Now of course, it is accepted as a very powerful custom. There have been many times that Native women have travelled long miles to be at a sacred ceremony only to find that their period has come on and that means disempowerment and exclusion.

It has been my experience of more than thirty years, and from discourse with women from coast to coast, that, for all practical purposes, the institution of the menstrual hut as a place where women pass on our ancient knowledge is not a reality for most Native women. Menstruation is a time of confusion, isolation, and fear. Many of the teachings have been lost because most of our mothers and grandmothers went away to residential boarding schools. It was a common practice years ago for Native children to leave home between the ages of six and eight. Often children saw their families only during the summer, or not at all, for years at a time. This practice cut the children off from their cultural roots, forcing them to take on many of the values and problems of European culture.

From the nuns, Native girls learned to read and write, to cook and sew, but they also learned to adopt the nuns' basic negative attitude towards being a woman. These feelings of shame and fear still haunt most Native women today, even though attendance at boarding schools has, for the most part, been abandoned in favour of local schooling.

As our ancient women's lore has faded, the teaching by Native medicine men has come to be dominant. Nowadays, there are a variety of medicine men on the "Holy Man Circuit" and very few Native women. The teachings these men offer are good, but they are basically for men. In the area of women's power and women's Blood, their information can be harmful or, at best, misleading. It is my own personal bias that men should teach men and women should teach women. Power struggles and sexual manipulation are so common between the male teacher and female student that, unless consciously controlled, this sexual energy gets in the way of learning.

To give an example of misleading information, I was twenty when I was told, by more than one medicine man, that I could not use, or even touch, my sacred objects during my period. I agonized each month about what to do. Should I take my things out of the house before I Bled? Could I keep them in the house but not touch them? Would they be safe? Or should I follow my intuition and use them anyway?

I was not alone. Other women whom I asked for guidance were just as confused as I. Men seemed so afraid of my Blood that I finally decided that if they wanted to stay away, then fine, but this was my Blood and these objects were my sacred things, so why shouldn't I use them when I wanted to?

Nevertheless, it took me many years and a lot of prayer to realize that I am a woman and must accept and use all my gifts as the Earth Mother intended. I am neither ashamed nor afraid of my Blood. My medicine tools stay with me whatever time of the month it is, and I use them whenever I need to, because they are for me, and their purpose is for my spiritual growth.

I still respect other people's rights to believe what they choose. I will not go to a ceremony given by someone else during my Moon time, not because I feel I am dangerous or unclean, but because I respect another person's right to believe as they choose. I am not going to push my beliefs on others. If I go to a ceremony and my period comes on, I will go away and set up a Moon Lodge. I will invite other women to come visit, to talk and share what has been revealed to me and what I have learned for myself by being in touch with my own body and the Mother Earth.

⟨∾⟩

C.N.S., TEACHER IN her late 40's; Victoria, BC

In our culture there is no time given for women to rest at the time of their periods. I think having such a retreat would make a big difference to a lot of women. Probably most of the PMS we experience in this culture is a direct result of no rest period at this time. Women's lib doesn't help with their big push to be just like a man.

⟨∾⟩

M., TEACHER IN HER 30's; Victoria, BC

It wasn't until I was eighteen or so, after I'd been menstruating for about seven years, that I finally clued in to what having a period really meant. It was a revelation at the time. I had read *Our Bodies, Ourselves* a couple years earlier (around 1978), so it wasn't as though I was growing up without the benefit of the liberated sixties behind me, but somehow I was so abstracted from my femaleness that I had retained the information on an intellectual level and had not translated it into "body knowledge." I didn't really connect with the process in my body.

I knew all the clinical aspects of my anatomy and, as a separate detail, I knew that love-making could result in pregnancy unless you protected yourself. I wasn't ignorant of the facts; I just hadn't made the connection.

Then, one day as I was sitting on the toilet feeling the Blood flow out of me, it suddenly hit me that what was Bleeding out of me could have become a baby, a part of my womb, and that the whole process would repeat itself, month after month. The sheer magic and power of this left me awed and trembling. For the first time I realized my period was something powerful and wonderful. Instead of seeing it as a drag, I felt strong and empowered. My Blood, flowing without need of wound, magically flowing and disappearing again without any violence committed, was a glory and a triumph to me.

I remember this as a special day; my body glorious in this Blood flow and I glorious in it. It still took many more years before I could resolve my feelings and accept my body totally and without reserve, respecting, loving, admiring it, honouring its beauty and magic and power, feeling proud of my womanness.

MOON, A TRAVELLING woman in her 50's

I take time off from the world almost every time I'm Bleeding. I just stop my activities and don't go out. When my son was living with me I didn't feel comfortable with him or his friends around. I felt very secretive about the fact that I was Bleeding. I didn't feel comfortable with male energy. Now he is older, and I can have my own space.

I used to feel uncomfortable washing out my Blood cloths in laundromats, so now I rinse them first, then wash them with my clothes. I used to feel sensitive with men around to watch, but now I feel it is my life and my Blood and if they have any problems with what I'm doing with these cloths, it's their problem, not mine.

B.S., WITCH IN HER 30's; rural Washington State

I enjoy being a pagan, and one of the most enjoyable things about being a pagan for me is the openness everyone feels about their bodies and bodily cycles. This is a totally new and refreshing feeling for me, so different from how I was raised. Let me give you an example.

About a month ago, I attended a two day pagan ceremony for Samhain. During the ceremony one of the women was called to the phone. She was listening to someone talking and I kept hearing her trying to urgently cut in. Finally she just handed the phone to a man nearby and rushed to the bathroom, leaving a trail of Blood behind her. I don't remember exactly what was said, but the Blood was openly acknowledged with love and laughter. There were comments jokingly made about where the trail might lead but nothing mean was said. It was very obvious that both the men and women present saw the whole thing as a natural event; something to celebrate rather than to ignore or be embarrassed about. Even when the woman came back to the phone, she wasn't upset. I thought to myself how very different this incident would have been if this had been in a Christian gathering. The Bleeding woman would have been totally humiliated, probably gone home in tears, while everyone who witnessed her shame would have tried to ignore the Blood on the floor, or quickly clean it up without comment.

To treat the event openly and humorously as a celebration of a magical event was a revelation for me. I value this body openness in pagan circles and, especially, many women's willingness to be open about their Blood with pagan men. I used to think before I came to the Craft that there was no hope for men; they were all losers. Now, through Wicca, I've met some very special men who can honour me as a woman and rejoice with me in my growing power. Disregarding personal sexual preferences in sacred space, I feel the need to balance the energies of the cosmos. So I do appreciate our pagan men's attitudes.

⚬≈⚬

J.N., MUSIC TEACHER in her late 40's; Victoria, BC

I've made a point about being really open with our kids about nudity and naturalness in the home so I've made no effort to hide my pads. It was after the summer solstice that it struck me that my sons wouldn't know about the wonders of menstruation and the really magical part of it. I think, having seen my pads, they only knew the disgusting part of my menstruation. It smells, and looks kind of bad because it is Blood, and you associate Blood with injury or pain or something bad. They didn't know or understand the wonderful part of menstruation and can never experience the ability to have a baby and re-create life. I decided to share this experience with them. They really responded in a positive way, especially my older son. He could see how that would be really important to me.

At university, I stayed in the dorms and there was one young girl who had really heavy periods, and all her friends would come and look after her. There were usually four or five of them, and I remember seeing her lying in bed, with all the others looking after her all night. I wasn't really part of the group, but I thought that the girl was lucky to have caring friends. I thought how menstruation bound us together as women. I didn't realize this until recently, but the nature tradition of women going off to a separate hut because it was a taboo was probably a gift to the women. It was time to get off alone, just be with women, and have those few days together meditating, away from the men. It was probably quite a moving experience. There are times when I would like to do that. I think it's a natural urge to run away when you have your period. Women get into trouble when they pretend everything is the same and act like a man; go to work, take your briefcase, ignore your cramps.

C.W., MOTHER AND HOUSEWIFE in her 20's; Winnipeg, MB

I took a trip with my son when he was four. We had just returned, and I was in the bedroom unpacking (with his help) when the doorbell rang. The only thing left in the suitcase was a plastic bag with some sanitary pads in it. I left them in the suitcase and went to answer the door. An old friend whom I hadn't seen for a while was calling. We got to talking and went to the kitchen to have tea. As we talked, I heard my son call me from the bedroom a few times, but I didn't pay much attention. I just called back that I'd finish unpacking later. His calling continued, but I ignored it and went on with my visit.

Finally, a very disgusted four-year-old marched into the kitchen holding a pad in each hand. You forgot your Pampers, Mom, he announced. Well, my friend and I started laughing. My son looked puzzled; he must have thought we were crazy, but it was quite funny. When I could control myself, I thanked him, gave him a drink, and went on with my visit.

B.W., STUDENT IN HER 20's; Toronto, ON

My brother was the youngest in a family of four girls. We were quite open about our periods around him when he was about three or four. We were expecting company one Christmas, and he wanted to help prepare for the big event. He was so small there wasn't much he could do, but he kept bugging us and getting in the way. Finally, my mother told him to set the table in the dining room, and to be sure and put a napkin at each place. Later, when we brought in the food, we had to laugh because he had put neatly by each plate a Kotex napkin. Fortunately, the guests were still in the living-room, so we had time to fix his mistake.

S.D., FARMER IN HER 40's; Aldergrove, BC

I'm so glad they have the stick-on kind of napkin now with the super deluxe sizes and the smaller ones for before and after. I remember using three at a time with those horrid belts that were always coming unadjusted and leaking all over the bloody place.

M.M., WITCH AND WRITER in her 50's; rural BC

When I had my period as a girl I was not allowed to use tampons in case they got lost inside. The big bulky pads that were available chafed the inside of my thighs until they were raw and bloody. It was impossible to wear pants over them.

M., TEACHER IN HER 30's; Victoria, BC

My quest for a perfect means of catching my Blood was finally resolved when I discovered sea-sponges – a real gift from Venus. I always think of her rising from the waves, her hand cupping the mound of her cunt, knowing our needs and giving us this sponge that grows in, of all things, the ocean waters.

J.Z.N., PSYCHIC READER in her 40's; Victoria, BC

For convenience sake, I use pads. I have a heavy flow, so unless I am going to stay at home, I have to use a pad along with a sponge, so why bother?

I am very upset about tampons. I just feel terrible that women use them. Most of them contain blood clotting agents. I realize, after many years, that the actual tissue of the uterus lining sheds in menstruation. I wonder about it coming away in the uterus of women using tampons and what effect these blood clotting agents have on the organs.

Some women want to ignore their periods, and if their flow isn't too heavy, tampons are convenient. I'm concerned, however, about the long term health effects of these products. These internally worn, chemically permeated substances must have some effect. I would think over time, say twenty years, the accumulation of the chemicals must be quite substantial.

If only we could design comfortable pads. I love the idea of reusable ones, but rags or old sheets somehow don't do it for me. I talked with a friend one day who made an interesting point. How can we bring women to really appreciate the sacrament of menstruation if we make and use disposable products, telling them this is bodily waste?

L.D., WITCH IN HER 20's; New York, NY

My Blood is sacred. I make my own pads – I don't want to kill trees or support men's industries like Kotex.

STARHAWK, AUTHOR AND witch; San Francisco, CA

There was a woman in the Reclaiming Collective who used to save her menstrual Blood, dry it in a saucer in the sun, then pound it up in a mortar and pestle. It would then be useful for spells. For a while, people involved in political action got into it, pouring Blood onto places like nuclear weapons plants. At one time, four of us poured Blood over the sign that is right across from Livermore Labs. The men used regular blood, the women used their menstrual Blood. This Blood had been gathered for a previous action that never happened, and had been saved in the freezer.

MOON, A TRAVELLING woman in her 50's

When I was living in the country, I didn't catch my Blood. I allowed it to flow free, which was always interesting to the children. I used to explain to the really little ones that I wasn't cut; this was what happened when my body didn't make a baby. This was the way my body let go of the special little bed it makes for babies inside the womb. They would always be very relieved to know I wasn't hurt.

When I do catch my Blood, it is a whole different thing. I went through a whole evolution of what to do. This evolutionary process actually started when I was living in Mexico about ten years ago. While I was there I found out that regular tampons (they didn't have supers) cost three times what they do in the States. This made me angry because many Mexican women look at the US as having a better way of life when maybe we don't. The only women who could get tampons were the young women who had gotten a job in a store or as a secretary or waitress. My anger and fear was that the women who bought the tampons would be separated from their mothers and sisters and that they would be ashamed of their Blood and their Blood cloths.

It was then that I started on the path of using blessed Blood cloths. I made my first Blood cloths out of dark red cotton velour. They were the same size as regular sanitary napkins. I filled them with what I thought would be absorbent materials like cottons and wools. I also made some tampons out of a sponge covered with velour and long braided strings. I made a bag out of the same cotton to carry them in. On the outside of the bag, I embroidered a picture of the uterus, ovaries, and fallopian tubes-the whole blessed reproductive system.

When I went to Mexico the next time, all this seemed too bulky to carry. That was the time I started using sponges to catch my Blood. I would only use a natural sponge as I had been to a factory where sponges were made – bleached and whitened with unnameable chemicals. Another concern about using sponges is that they come from a highly polluted area of the Mediterranean Sea. If you use a sponge I would suggest a three part purification process. When you begin Bleeding, first wash the sponge in water that has been boiled but let to cool to lukewarm. Next, let it soak in a tea of herbs beneficial to the vagina like plantain or mugwort. The third part of the process is to sun dry the sponge for a few hours. At the end of my period, I repeat the same process and put the sponge away in a bag that won't allow dust or free floating bacteria to land on it.

When I was living in Mexico, I found using a sponge to be very convenient. With my lover's help I could even change it travelling on the buses. She would block the view by sitting in the aisle seat while I took out my sponge, wrung it out in a little bowl I carried, rinsed it with water a few times, and put it back in. Then I would throw the water and Blood out the window without anyone noticing.

When I returned to the United States, I started using Blood cloths again and I've been using the same kind for the last eleven years. I use old sheets to make my cloths. They are very precious to me and very well washed. I don't like to use new cotton around any opening of my body, because new cottons are so permeated with poisons.

I tear my sheets into strips that are wide enough to fold over a good-sized sanitary pad. I use different thicknesses of pad as I Bleed. I don't wear underpants as I can't bear to have anything binding my waist and thighs. I tie a belt around my waist that is about an inch wide. Then I lay out the strip of sheeting, which is about six to eight inches wide and almost two feet long. In the centre of the sheeting, I place a little pillow or pad made of absorbent materials. I fold the sheet strip over the pad twice and place the pad next to my vulva. I bring the ends of the sheet up to my waist and tuck them over the belt allowing the ends to hang down on the inside. Then I pin them in place. I put the tails inside so that when I'm naked it looks like a loin cloth. I have a red corduroy bag now that I keep my Blood cloths in. When I finish my Bloods, I rinse out my cloths in water so I can give the water to plants. Even as a travelling woman, I do this no matter where I am.

Recently I was away from my cloths when I started to Bleed. I had to use a paper pad and I found it scratchy and uncomfortable. I won't use tampons because I don't trust the corporations and what they put in them, so my Blood cloths and I will keep company until I make the passage into menopause. I won't regret its coming, but I don't wish for it either because I like my Bloods.

One way I have used my Blood cloths is in political work. When I've been at military bases, I've taken my Blood cloths and tied them on the gates. I've often tied the gates shut with a Blood cloth and, when I do, I like it to be a really Bloody cloth. I Bleed very heavily for two days and spread the Blood out well so it is really visible. I think it's appropriate because I feel war is menstrual envy. Men shedding their blood and other people's blood is their way of menstruating and feeling strong and powerful. It is amazing that as much pride as men carry, and as much patriotic admiration they get for wounding each other and making blood flow, these same men are absolutely stunned and repulsed by women's Blood and by a Blood cloth being tied on the fence. Where I've done this, the men usually take the cloth off by cutting it. When I was at Greenham Common in England, no one touched the cloths, and each month I put a fresh one on the gate. One time the men teased me about why I should want to close the gates instead of trying to get in there with them. When I told them I was tying it shut with my Blood cloth, there was stunned silence. No one touched the cloth.

When I was at Seneca, I had to change my cloth, so I went across the street from the base where some cars were and changed my Blood cloth behind a vehicle. There were some counter-demonstrators there, and an older woman started yelling and complaining that I was peeing on the Earth. When I explained to her that I was only changing my Blood cloth, she said it was even worse, especially doing it in front of a twelve-year-old girl. I asked her what was so terrible about that and said that, if the girl hasn't already Bled, she would Bleed very soon, and that it really wasn't so awful to Bleed. We went through quite a long discussion, but this woman did not cease to be repulsed by my having been public with my Blood.

Another time, when I was in Europe, I massaged an Irish woman. As I worked, she asked me if it was true that women were throwing their menstrual pads into the base. I knew she was upset about it, so my reply was vague. I knew that no matter what I said, this woman's response would be the same as the Seneca woman's response. Some women were even repulsed when I did a blessed Blood cloth show at Land in New Mexico. It was women's land, a Leo party, and it seemed a wonderful time to be with the wind and the fire. Blood seemed appropriate at the time, and I had Blood cloths of mine with beautiful patterns on them. I asked other women for their cloths, hung up a clothes line, and pinned on these cloths.

Some of the women were just ecstatic and happy and thought it was a wonderful idea. They looked like a beautiful painting. Other women thought it was absolutely disgusting, repulsive, and gross.

⚜

MARGOT ADLER, AUTHOR; New York, NY

In 1966, I was in jail for twenty days at the Santa Rita Women's prison in California. It was for sitting in, in 1964, at Sproul Hall at the University of California during the free speech movement. In jail, none of the women were allowed to have tampons. We were told that it was because it caused a security problem. Women could pass messages in the tampons when they left or entered jail. So I learned an art form that I have never seen or heard of anywhere else. Women would teach each other this trick. One Kotex or Modess pad equals two tampons. We would sit on our cots and roll these, just as in the 60's we might have rolled joints. You take the Kotex and cut it in half at the middle. Then you unroll the gauze and lay it out as a square. Then you roll the inside up small into a little roll, put the gauze around it, as if you were wrapping a bottle of wine, and you make a knot at the end. The result is two tampons for each Kotex. I still remember sitting on my cot in jail and rolling myself twenty-four tampons from a box of twelve Kotex ... they worked well, by the way.

⚜

B.S.C., WITCH IN HER 20's; Chicago, IL

A friend of mine told me she knew a woman who leaves Bloodied sanitary napkins on the seat of her car, on her bicycle handlebars, or on the bedroom window ledge to discourage anyone from taking her stuff. When I first heard this I was shocked and a little disgusted. Then, as I thought about it, the idea sort of grabbed me, and I could see the sense in it. In some ways, it is really right on and it just might work.

Most men, no matter what their race, culture, economic, or educational background are disgusted by, and perhaps a little bit frightened by, menstrual

Blood. Tell me, sisters, who are responsible for most of the stolen cars, B & E's, rapes, and murders in the world? Men are. So, maybe it could make a difference in your protection to declare your space and your possessions with your Blood.

A women in my coven had her store broken into. I told her how to use her Blood to protect her space. We got to talking and decided the women in our group could donate enough pads and tampons to make mobiles for the doors and windows. Each night, we could hang them up after closing and each month we could renew them. We had a bjt of nervous giggling about it and that was all, but maybe, if it happens again, well ...

I think it takes courage to question and go against such strong rooted taboos in our culture and be so radical with menstrual Blood. I myself haven't had an occasion to use this powerful medicine of protection. I don't own a car or live in a high crime area but, if the need arises, I would use my Blood with no hesitation in this way.

⚬≫≪

B.E.S., POLITICAL ACTIVIST and witch in her late 20's; BC

I have a friend who has become very active in the environmental movement to stop clear-cutting our forests. She has talked to me about her frustrations with some of the political actions planned where male egos and the deliberate use of violent, confrontational tactics appear to do more harm than help. We are both very concerned and feel that the environmental movement is doomed to failure if it continues to rely on, and use, these dominating, power battling, violent male tactics.

To create a new world, we must begin by using a new structure to achieve not only this goal, but others as well. We feel women need to become more involved in the movement, not just by following male leaders, but by acting in our women's way, adding our rituals and our Moon Blood to our political activities.

Over the past few months, I've watched my friend change. At one point, she went alone into the forests of Vancouver Island. She fasted, prayed, and received a spirit guide. She opened herself up enough so that she could communicate directly with the big trees. This is quite amazing, she says. This wasn't her life-style before this experience.

Many of the more political/scientific types in the movement still don't take her seriously, and think she's a real nut. Nevertheless, this intuitive, psychic, woman-like communication with the Earth and other beings of the Earth is actually just what we should be trying to achieve. Rather than violence, she hopes to use ritual drama and street theatre as more effective tools to help change public attitudes. This isn't the whole answer, but it's a start.

I've also suggested to her the ritual use of Moon Blood as part of political action. Imagine a logging road in the bush, bulldozers at the ready when, along with the regular protesters, thirty or fifty women arrive in bloodied skirts, their faces painted with their Moon Blood, wailing and chanting and tying their Blood cloths on the old trees as an act of love and protection. With their woman's power, they would offer rituals for the protection of our Earth Mother and the trees. This would be a very powerful act.

If we connect with our bellies to the Earth Mother, if we feel it within and open ourselves to the trees and the Earth, we will be guided on how to save our planet. It is time that we women came forward to reclaim our power and use our sacred Blood and our woman's wisdom to heal and save the Earth.

❦

AN INTERVIEW WITH JEAN Mountaingrove, teacher, menstrual lodge facilitator and workshop instructor in her 50's; rural Oregon

I have been interested in menstruation for a number of years, but it is only since I got through with my second Saturn Return that I've been able to focus my energies again around what I consider to be my present heart path. Someone questioned why a post-menopausal woman is so interested in menstruation. My only explanation can be that I feel it's an assignment from the Goddess; that it was given to me, not that I chose it. To me, the way in which I'm carrying out this task is typically Crone in that I'm doing it for the larger community. I'm doing it to change our culture. I think those larger concerns of culture and community are quite appropriately Crone areas of concern, interest, and work.

As I thought about menstruation, as I wondered what to do with it, I worked on intuition and went where I was drawn. In the winter, which is my most intuitive time, I did some meditations with a spirit guide I call Womb-Woman. I was given a meditation and a guided visualization in which the journey through our internal organs is experienced without using any medical terms for any parts of our body.

I experienced it as very beautiful, very mysterious, and totally perfect, and I feel that this meditation has been very energizing for the many women who have experienced it. The visualization could also be used diagnostically; if a woman were experiencing any difficulty in her menstrual cycle, she could take this journey and, if she were intuitively tuned in, be able to identify the places where the energy was blocked or where things were in need of healing or re-alignment. I haven't yet had an experience with that, but it seems to be a possibility. We could do our own internal psychic diagnosis, identify the problems, and maybe deal with them psychically through meditation on internal structures and processes in a very loving fashion.

I also started doing menstrual huts. I've done five huts at five different women's gatherings. I had no exact ideas about what I was going to do. I just collected everything red that I could get my hands on. Each time I'm given a different kind of space, and each time I simply do whatever comes to me intuitively with what is offered in that space.

Other women seem to react to the hut in a very positive fashion. I don't have any particular awareness of goal in making menstrual huts except to lead women to experience Bleeding as beautiful and spiritual. I have no preconceptions about what they do with their space. I feel it should be available to all women, Bleeding or not, simply because we have all been denied the experience of our menstrual periods being treated as beautiful and sacred. I can imagine in a long term menstrual space there would be different times for women who are Bleeding, and other times for pre-menstrual women, and still other times for Crones, but I don't feel that the kind of work I do needs those distinctions. I think, coming out of my Croneness, that I'm more concerned about the affecting all women's attitudes towards menstruation rather than particularly honouring the one who is, at that moment, Bleeding.

From the beginning, I began to get complaints from women who had hysterectomies: They were feeling left out. Of course I was disturbed – I didn't want any woman to feel left out, as I feel having a womb is the basic definition of what a female is. I thought this emphasis on menstruation and our reproductive process would be unifying, and that all women all over the world, of all ages, could identify and feel included. That is what woman is – she is womb.

So, when women with hysterectomies came to me and said they felt they couldn't come to the meditation or the menstrual sanctuary, I had to come up with an answer, and this came to me very quickly. Once we have had a physical womb, we always bear the psychic imprint; we always have the aura, the energy body of a womb. Women can always relate to that intuitively and psychically even without a physical womb.

I have begun to think more about menstruation. I didn't want any negative things associated with menstruation at all. The idea of a cleansing through menstruation comes out of the idea that women are unclean and need to be cleansed. I didn't want to give any energy to that sort of concept. Menstruation is a process that is cyclical, that repeats itself, and the process has to do with life-giving and creativity, not cleansing. When the egg is absorbed in my menstrual meditation, I don't know if there is a discharge. I did some anatomy study to try to learn more about the process. Physiologically, I think that the egg is discharged, but in my meditation, and what I believe to be spiritually true, is that the life energy of the egg is reabsorbed into the uterus. Therefore, I use the symbolism of the egg dissolving into electrical energy. This is represented as a shooting star. That energy permeates the uterus and is a creative life force energy for the woman's use.

Then I began to deal with the purpose of this cycle. The Goddess would not create us in this beautiful universe, in which every bit of the ecological system helps every other bit, without there being some purpose.

Again the answer came intuitively. These periods are a time of withdrawal and inner focus and peace, not a time of doing, not an external. I stayed with that a while and then it occurred to me that this is a time for developing our psychic and intuitive strengths and abilities. I read that one of the characteristics of a menarchial girl is increased daydreaming. It seemed to me this was a mark of growing intuitive focus, imagination, and psychic development. It occurred to me the term period means periods of opportunity, recurring opportunities to contact our inner wise selves through our psychic and intuitive openness at this time. So, I just playfully labelled them training periods in which we could gradually increase our confidence, our skill and our ease of trusting our intuitive understanding. If at that time we have this intuitive awareness, and we then absorb the egg with its creative energy, then we express that. Each month we say we were given more intuitive awareness and the ability to express it. If this were to recur through our lives almost four hundred times, think what powerfully, centred, intuitive, wise beings we would be if we had utilized all these opportunities.

As well, we have been drawn deeply into ourselves, and released over and over again, every twenty-eight to thirty days. We have done whatever we needed to do in the world in terms of discovering our competence through what we do and make. Then we are given the Goddess's blessing, freed from this monthly change. She says:

Now go forth daughters, old women, and use this in terms of long range planning. You are not going to be taken down deep inside yourself each month. You are going to have a whole year! You can now take your wisdom and stretch it out over a long span of planning. You can trust your energy to be there month after month. I expect big things from you.

And that is the time we should be able to take this wisdom and skill and plan big things for ourselves, our communities, our people.

I know that in my own life I have become a solar cycle person in which my best intuitive times are January through March. This is the equivalent, in a yearly cycle, of the pre-menstrual period-before the spring, before the re-birth of that youthful energy.

I feel that the kind of wisdom that we need we can always rediscover through this inner psychic alertness. Men's knowledge has to be learned from someone else and it might get lost; but I don't believe women's wisdom can ever be lost. I believe that the psychic knowledge can be obtained through our periods and that it is the same knowledge that ancient women knew.

Our knowledge of the universe and the world as it is, about the reality of our bodies, of the stars, and of our inner beings is timeless.

They can never destroy what we need to know. Our wisdom for the nurturance of life, the preservation of life, is always available. I believe the Mother planned it so we could never destroy that; it would always be available to us. That's very thrilling to me because I've always felt connected to very ancient women although I didn't know why. I didn't know what it was. Now I know that it is through my womb, through my cycles, that I've turned to the same place and it has always been the same place. That's the heart of it.

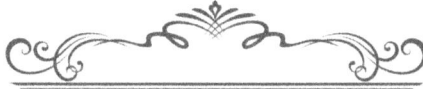

Blood Tides

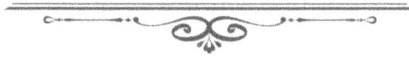

Self-revelation

LIKE THE TIDES OF THE ocean
  My body's one with the moon
  Both creation and destruction
  Are the blessings of my womb.
  C.W.

OVER THE CENTURIES, styles of beauty have changed in patriarchal cultures around the world. At various times, rounded bellies, curvy hips, full breasts, or slim waists have all been considered the ideal of beautiful womanhood. What has not changed throughout the centuries has been women's dissatisfaction with whatever bodily features they may possess. The beautiful woman as well as the plain one is never quite content with her lot in life.

This lack of self-worth and love exhibited by most women has a lot to do with the cultural teachings we accept as truths. Unfortunately, these truths all too often get transformed into patterns of emotional and physical illness and disease, particularly in highly industrialized societies around the world. The last thirty years has seen a shift to the thinner ideal of female beauty. Fashion, and dieting products and services have become big money making operations. These commercial enterprises capitalize on the modern woman's insecurities about herself. Somewhere, in a dark corner of our minds, is the alluring fantasy fostered by the media that if we could only look a certain way all our dreams would come true. However, a woman's dreams turn into nightmares as the stress of trying to conform to this ideal often ruins her health. Today women who thirty years ago would have been considered sickly or malnourished are the models of beauty for young women. Many health care professionals are becoming alarmed. New studies are linking extreme thinness to a variety of health problems including menstrual irregularities and pain, childbirth complications, osteoporosis, and even premature death.

Many ancient religions around the world teach us that the belly (or in the case of a woman, the womb) is the seat of power. The belly is the spiritual as well as physical centre that unites us to the universe. Through our bellies, we are grounded in this most physical of realities. Through our bellies, we can hear the voice of our universal higher power speak to us. Through our bellies we become one with the living Earth, Herself.

Most of us have been taught to suck in our bellies and hold them tight. This action, over time, numbs our awareness of our whole pelvic region. We lose touch with our self-hood and with the spirit within. We become easily controlled by others and influenced by their will. As women, there is a need for much healing to take place in our lives, both collectively and individually. We can begin this process of opening up by increasing our awareness of our bodies (especially in the belly) and of our link with all life.

In this chapter, women share some insights and revelations about their bodies, their periods, and sexuality.

⌾≫

L.B., TRAPPER IN HER 50's; Yukon Territory

When I used to go to the Indian dances up North, I used to feel so good. All the men of my age (forties) and older would flirt with me. I never lacked a partner. Those skinny white girls sat on the side at Indian dances, not me. Indians, like most indigenous people around the world, like fatter women. In the old days I guess people who had a little extra weight found it easier to make it through hard times. I'm not sure why but big women are valued all over the world except here in North America.

Our young people have it much harder. Movies and T.V. are giving them different images to live by. It's very sad to see the young girls hating themselves in a way their mothers and grandmothers never did. Maybe this body image problem is why so many more young Native girls drink than when I was young.

H.P., WITCH IN HER 50's; Chicago, IL

Over forty years ago, when I was a young girl, I can remember my mother commenting that a beautiful woman was supposed to be plump enough that when she wore a bathing suit, you couldn't see daylight between her thighs. That is not to say that she would be fat; just that she looked like a woman with full breasts, curvy hips and rounded, tapering legs. As I've grown older, I've watched the image of the ideal beautiful woman grow thinner and thinner. Nowadays, the ideal is a pretty face, flat chest, no hips, and skinny thighs. To rob a woman of the things that make her a woman is to rob her of her woman's power. Without breast and belly, hips and thighs, she is nothing; not a man nor woman but a weak nothing person with no mind of her own.

I think men who encourage their women to look like this are afraid of strong, powerful women. They are really homosexual deep down and if they want someone who looks like that they should go find a young boy and be done with it, instead of laying their perversions onto women.

M.H., STUDENT IN HER late 20's; Los Angeles, CA

I like big women who look like real women. If most men are threatened and don't like it, that's just fine by me because it leaves more women for a righteous dyke like me.

K., DANCER IN HER 30'S; New Orleans, AL

I recognize that stress is particularly responsible for my weight, but instead of feeling bad or going on crash diets to lose, I'll accept who I am and love who I am right now. A couple years ago I started a physical fitness program. I did aerobics four times a week and swam two to three times.

I didn't lose weight, to my amazement, but I felt good. I also began to dance again, something I let slide as my family demanded more of my time. Last year, I began to teach belly dancing again. It felt good when I danced, especially at pagan rituals. I feel the power of the Mother moving in me and through me. I feel totally connected to the Earth at such times.

I would encourage any woman to take up belly dancing. It is one of our ancient rituals and very sacred. For me, though, it's not the folk art, or the choreography, but the feeling in your body that is important. That's how I teach my classes. It is the feeling, the way your body moves and experiences life that counts, not the sterile form of a dance where you take two steps forward and two back, twist, twist, and so on. That type of dance has its place, but it's not my way. I encourage large women to come to my classes. We need to experience our selves as beautiful, loving beings, and for me, the Old Religion and the belly dance are the keys to a new way of living. Beside, you have to have a belly if you want to be a good belly dancer, right?

⚜

J.Z.N., PSYCHIC READER in her 40's; Victoria, BC

When I hit sixteen, I was 140 pounds at 5'6". Up until then I had always been much thinner and was criticized for being too thin. At that time, I felt as good as I possibly could about my body considering the feedback I got from the people around me. I was always told I was horrific, ugly, and that no one would ever want me. The ironic thing, coming from a family of heavy women, was that when I got to 140 pounds I remember my mother telling me I had better watch my weight. I found this ironic because all my life they had been at me for being so thin. It didn't seem to make any sense whatsoever. I promptly lost fifteen pounds. There were a lot of vague issues around my weight. I knew I didn't want to gain too much weight, but I never looked closely as to why. Finally, in therapy, it came out specifically in relation to my father, who prefers heavy women. His attitude towards women was that they were stupid but that he couldn't do without them. Getting to that point in therapy I promptly lost ten pounds and I didn't have a lot to lose. I basically stopped eating. I had no appetite. When I dropped the weight so suddenly my therapist told me to eat lots of protein or people would think I was becoming anorexic.

I realized that in working through my relationship with my father, I wanted him to see me as a person, not as an object to be used. I didn't want him to categorize me in the same way he categorized other women. This was my reason for always being thin.

❧

H.C., PSYCHOLOGIST in her 30's; Los Angeles, CA

I was part of a women's new Moon Circle gathering. It was a group of Jewish women. In this tradition, the new moon is a sacred day called Rosh Chodesh (new month). Each month the Hebrew calendar begins with the new moon. We met in various configurations as a group for several years, our work taking the form of sharing and exploring the focus of that season, that month, in terms of our own inner, spiritual loves, women's expressions in dance, music, chanting etc.

Within six months of working together, all the group members (eight or nine) had shifted in their menstrual cycles so that all of us were in the time of our Blood flow when we gathered at the new moon. Subsequent new members joined our rhythm in this same way.

❧

C.S., WITCH IN HER 30's; Dallas, TX

I think there are two kinds of women: the Ovulators and the Bleeders. Ovulators peak their energies around the time of possible conception, while Bleeders' energies peak at menstruation. I'm not sure if it is universal, but the women I know who fall into these two categories are often quite different in temperament. Ovulators (and that is most women) have menstrual cramps. They are nurturing to others and not themselves. At least they think they must be nurturing the sort of image of the good Catholic wife and mother. You know, the breeder and good wife and martyr. I grew up with that crap so forgive me if I'm bitter. That type of life-style is not for me. I saw what it did to my mother, ten children, and an old woman at forty-five, always at my father's beck and call. That's an Ovulator for you.

On the other hand, a Bleeding woman is different. She enjoys her body in all it's cycles. She is more self-assured and comfortable with both men and women. She is usually very creative and able to nurture herself as well as others. I guess I'm a bit biased on the subject, but I do think my basic premise is valid. There are two peaks of energy in a woman's cycle and she chooses, either consciously, or by cultural design, to attune herself to one of these energy flows. That energy flow, in turn, affects how she lives her life. Think about it and you will find I am right.

⚜

C.W., WITCH AND HOMESTEADER in her 30's; rural New Mexico

I've been paying attention to my cycle for a few years. Now I keep a diary and from that I can tell my cycle goes something like this. When my period comes, I feel good but lazy. I want to relax, read, do creative things with my mind, but nothing too physical. I have, however, led some very powerful rituals while Bleeding. Sometimes they were very physically demanding, like dancing all night. Though I've done this, I prefer doing ritual just before my period rather than after I've started because I really do want to take it easy, at least for the first few days when my flow is heaviest.

After my flow has ceased, I go through a real down time for three or four days. I get depressed and very emotional though not like the raw intenseness that I can feel if I'm upset during my flow. This post-Bleeding time is just a sadness when the day to day routine gets to be a real drag.

I know when I'm ovulating because my fluids increase and I have a slight clear discharge from my vagina. My energy level is high. Physically it is time to go on an all day hike or camping trip. I feel good, but it's not a creative or emotional high for me. After ovulation, I also go through a three or four day slump, just like after I Bleed. I start picking up as I come closer to my period.

Two or three days before I Bleed is my ultimate energy peak for the month. This is an all around energy peak, creative and emotional as well as physical. In fact, my physical peak is probably higher at midcycle than premenstrual, but because my whole body, mind, and emotions are working together, it is an all-over high for me. I sing better, write more creatively, and do my best ceremonial work. When I Bleed, it is like the power is still on full tilt, but it shifts perspective from an outward directed to an inward directed channel. I really enjoy it. I've gone into as much detail as I have here because I want women to know that there are other ways of viewing our bodily cycles than the way we were taught to believe.

⚜

R.R., MOTHER AND PART-time secretary in her late 20's; Phoenix, AZ

At the full moon, I'm very active, but as my menses draws near, at the new moon, I become quieter and more withdrawn. I have been taught that when I Bleed, I, like all other women am most open to hear the spirit. I believe that. I know that I am very receptive and impressionable then, so as a protection, because I get very stressed out, I try to withdraw from the world and nurture myself. I read or draw or do other things that I enjoy. I clear away old stuff and try to make myself in tune to the Great Mystery.

I heard Brook Medicine Eagle speak once. She likened this time to the vision quest experience that men go through when they need guidance. She says that each month women have the opportunity to call for a vision from Mother Earth. Each month we are cleansed and renewed, and the dreams and visions that come to us at this time, we should take back to our communities for action. So, as the moon waxes, I become more active. Brook Medicine Eagle taught me that whatever we receive during our monthly Bleeding, we put out in the next phase as we move toward ovulation. This can be good or bad magnified outward. That is why I try to follow that natural cycle and it certainly has made a difference in my life. It's helped me to serve others in the world around me through my dreams and my actions.

⚜

C., WITCH IN HER 30'S; Oregon

Sexual religious rites, where you are going to use having sex for religious purposes, place a lot of restrictions on moon phase. The most commonly used rite of the Celtic tradition is the "Drawing down the Moon." This is a full moon/ ovulation phase rite which combines sword and wand (usually air and fire energy, or in less commonly used configurations, water and fire energy), magic, and usually ritual sex with your partner in magic. Many

Wiccans, gay and straight, use this ritual. It seems to work best when the woman, or two women (in the case of lesbians), are at mid-cycle and the moon is full.

Most women do not practice Dark Moon rituals. However, they are part of the Wiccan tradition. They are more powerful if you are Bleeding or about to do so. Ritual sex will often induce Bleeding.

Since most of us are cautious about believing every word of the Elders in traditions which have been suppressed, we think it best to experiment and record what happens. My experience is that when I'm in my moon I like to drift off into trance by myself or with a few others. I don't like to organize complicated ceremonies or dance all night. Sex is fine, producing some weird and wonderful trips; but you have to be careful with ritual sex to bring your partner back to normal consciousness. I've written some of my finest works the day before or the first day of my period.

I recommend taking a day off every month to honour one's cycle (a real test of respect for women). I would build a nice Moon hut to retreat to for meditation and use it regularly.

⚬⚬⚬

J.Z.N., PSYCHIC READER in her 40's; Victoria, BC

I'm really regular and if I'm two days out I get in a bit of a panic. My cycle alternates between twenty-four and twenty-eight days each month. At the time of my periods, I'm usually more intense. I'm very short tempered. I may crave affection, but as for sex, unless there is someone in my life, I can't afford to pay attention to it or I'll climb the walls. I have, in the past, noticed an increase of interest around menstruation and ovulation. I'm very seasonal. February is the worst time of the year for me. I go into heat. I am a spring baby and I wake up in February. It's very difficult for me to do any intellectual work at that time because I'm just too horny.

When women work or live together, their rhythms will synchronize. That doesn't mean they will all start on the same day, but it does mean that they will be clumped together at one end of the month. Another aspect is the sun/moon angle when you were born. There is a higher percentage of babies born around full moon so what it means is that these women will ovulate around the time of the full moon and then Bleed at new moon. Women, like myself, born at new moon, ovulate then and Bleed at the full moon. I find it very disruptive to live with women on the opposite cycle. I don't know what decides this shift. I think it is an unconscious consensus. It isn't because one women is stronger than another or the minority accommodating the majority. I don't know what it is, but I've watched it work for quite a few years.

I also know, from personal experience or observation, that your ovulation cycle can be affected by various circumstances such as stress or travel. You can ovulate twice in one cycle or even ovulate spontaneously if you are really into what you are doing with the person you are doing it with. This is a little scary – so much for the rhythm method. I have ovulated during my period and gotten pregnant so I know it does happen. Looking back, I realized that when I got pregnant it was the new moon which would normally have been my ovulation. At the time, I was close to other women whose cycles were different and I was in the process of shifting to their rhythms, so even though I was Bleeding, it was my natural ovulation time, so I got pregnant three days into my period.

⌾⚬⚬⚬⌾

K.F., TREE PLANTER; Victoria, BC

When I make love to the woman I love, it is like making love to Mother Earth herself. I've always had a strong, intimate connection with the natural world which has always felt like a strong female spirit-nurturing and giving, sensual, powerful, and creative. Until I pursued my lesbian nature, I went to Mother Earth to feel all those qualities in me. My Bleeding time often felt like an inconvenience and, initially, a disempowering time.

There were a few times that weren't like this. Once, when I was in the woods in the heat of the summer, I allowed my Blood to flow unimpeded onto the moss and soil. That was a very powerful time for me. I was alone, naked, and I didn't really know what compelled me to do it. There I was, looking at my Blood on the green moss – like an offering of life. I felt love from the Earth entering through my vagina, opened and relaxed. I felt very safe with Her.

That was just a hint of a different perspective for me, but I found when I started to connect with my power through doing this ritual, the feelings that came up were so strong that I became afraid and shut off the experience, just like a child caught doing something wrong.

Now I find myself in a loving relationship with a woman and I'm starting to connect with that power and passion again in a different yet very healing way. It is more than an exchange between two people. It feels like I am physically making love to Mother Earth as well. It is as though my partner is the beautiful female link to the beautiful female spirit of the Earth, Herself. For me, there is no separation and I am making love to both. I guess a part of me has always thought this, but now it is so much more real for me – I can really feel it.

Physically loving L. during her Blood was a deepening of this feeling for me. Before this experience, when I thought about what it would be like to make love to someone at this time of the month, I came face to face with how I felt about my own menstrual Blood, let alone anyone else's. I had always felt a level of revulsion while caring for my needs at this time of the month – the smell, the sight – I felt unclean. When I thought about tasting, touching, smelling, and being intimate with L. during her period, I had mixed feelings. Part of me pulled back from the experience, but just as I was drawn to Bleed in the woods, another part of me was drawn to being with her during this time.

It was the full moon both times that I made love to her during her Bleed. The first time she had just returned from spending a few hours at a women's Moon Lodge gathering. She felt so strong and sensual, my thoughts of revulsion dissolved as I was so physically, emotionally, and spiritually drawn to being sexual with her and she with me. L. was so open and receptive and beautiful; she smelled like deep, moist, iron rich Earth and tasted the same. It was intoxicating for me and a deep experience for the both of us.

⁂

C.J., TREE PLANTER in her 20's; Ontario

I had just gone off the pill about three months before I went tree planting. When I left, I still hadn't had a period. My doctor said it wasn't anything to worry about. It was interesting, however, that within a few weeks of being in camp, all the women there were having periods at more or less the same time. I still wasn't Bleeding, but I felt the same as when I was menstruating. My breasts would be tender and I would feel deeply emotional, but there was no Bleeding. I started to wonder if I might be pregnant (there was a possibility of this, despite what the doctor had said), especially when I started having the dreams about the little girl. These weren't sleeping dreams – they would come to me at any time. When you are doing a repetitive job like tree planting, your body does most of the work and you get into a rhythm. Only about two-and-a-half per cent of your mind is needed; the rest of it just drifts off somewhere.

It was just about three or four days before my period should have started when I began to have these vivid day dreams about the child. I'd be working alone and it would feel like someone was beside me. I could almost see her there, close by. The image would be so strong ... I would walk down the trail and she would be right there in the bushes beside me, stopping now and then to hold a branch out of my path. I got so I didn't want to work with anyone else on the crew because, when the others were nearby, she wouldn't come to me.

This was very powerful for me and, to this day, I'm not sure what the vision of her meant. I wondered if it was the child part of me or an unborn child in me; but whatever she was, I loved her very much.

Then I thought I would have to take a look at whether I wanted a child. I wasn't sure that I did. It took all my time and energy to take care of myself. Whatever it was I really don't know, but, after a few days, I started to Bleed.

I had gone on the pill in the first place because I had very bad cramps for years. The pill helped the cramps but after a while I decided I didn't want to take them anymore so I quit.

That night in the camp when the Bleeding started, it was the worst it had ever been. I was so sick, I couldn't even walk or see properly. The pain was so intense they finally had to take me to the hospital, where the doctor made me stay overnight. After that I went back to camp, by which time the doctor had convinced me to go back on the pill again.

Moreover, when I got back, within two days of that episode, every woman in camp began to Bleed again, even though it was only midcycle for most of them.

I stayed on the pill until about a month ago when I stopped taking them again. I don't want to take them, in spite of the cramps I may start having again. I haven't Bled yet so I don't know what will happen. But I plan to stay off them from now on, no matter what.

⚜

G.A., IN HER 40'S; Eva Beach, Hawaii

I'm an earth sign, a Taurus. I love the Mother Earth, She is a great being. I pray for this planet a lot, and, for some reason I can't explain, my body is very sensitive to the Earth's movements, like a seismograph. I can tell when an earthquake is going to happen, especially if the quake is to take place somewhere along the Pacific Rim. When the Earth begins to shift, the pain begins for me around my eyes, then it goes to my ears. If the shift is over water, I hear a sort of roaring in my ears. If the shift is over land, it sounds more like a ringing. As the movement intensifies, I get a bad migraine, then the pain travels down the back of my neck. If the symptoms continue, I get stomach cramps around my solar plexus. My whole body starts to ache. At this point I know the quake is going to be over 5.0 on the Richter scale. If the quake will be over 6.7, my period will come on along with the other symptoms. I could have two or more periods a month. The worst one I ever felt was a quake measuring 7.3, I was totally bed-ridden and I was so sick. When the symptoms begin, the quake is usually about five days away, but if the symptoms are more severe, or come on faster, I start eliminating days because it will come much faster and be stronger. When this happens I am so sick and no kind of medication can help me, so I just stay in bed and focus my prayer on helping the Mother Earth.

⚜

L.C., NURSE IN HER 30's; Nanaimo, BC

I used to have an underactive thyroid so I didn't start my periods until I was about sixteen. My periods started out very sporadically. This confused me as I never knew when to expect them nor why they were so irregular. I'd had a few bad experiences being out somewhere and starting to Bleed with no pads around so I started carrying a pad or two with me wherever I went.

When I was in college, I polled the girls in my dorm and found I wasn't so unusual. Many women, for one reason or another, have irregular cycles. In fact, only two girls in our whole dorm had a cycle lasting twenty-eight days. During that time, I went on the pill and this helped to regulate my cycle. I stayed on the pill for a number of years but lately, I have been worrying more and more about the side effects, so I think I'll stop.

⤬

K.P., POET AND MOTHER in her late 20's; Victoria, BC

When I was on the pill, I felt increasingly ill at ease. It took me about two years to realize that these were not periods I was having, these two drips and a drop that I didn't like. There is something cleansing and reassuring about taking part in that cycle that I missed when I was on the pill. As a kid when I heard the term "period," I envisioned it as a full stop; in other words, the sentences of my life are punctuated by my periods.

How do I feel during my cycle? About seventy-two hours before I start Bleeding I get a pre-menstrual hyper. I have a lot of energy, but it depends on how it is used. If I'm sitting on a lot of feelings, they tend to come up at that time. When I was trying to cope with a lot of anger, it would always come up. When nothing is upsetting in my life, it is just a hyper. When I actually start Bleeding, it's like coming into the autumn. It's a surge of real energy for me. I know that it's my time because, keeping a journal and a temperature chart as I used to, you can see the swell of my production of writings at the end of the month rather than in the middle of ovulation. It's quite well documented. It has helped me focus. My periods are not only the end of one cycle, but also the beginning of the next.

I think women in our culture have to work at viewing menstruation positively because, in our culture, we have so many more periods than other women around the world. We usually begin younger because of better nutrition and, with artificial means of birth control, women aren't pregnant or lactating all the time. This is why we must work so hard. There isn't a natural program for such a long sustained time of menstruating.

~⚬⚬~

Y., BOOKKEEPER; HELENA, MO

I haven't paid that much attention to my cycle, but since the question came up, I'd say I get really energized around the time of my ovulation. I can just go and go. Then when my period comes, I'm a real bitch. I get mean, crabby, and just leave me alone because if you don't, watch out!

~⚬⚬~

G., WAITRESS IN HER 40's; Holbrook, AZ

I get very depressed around my period. I feel all swollen and tender, and just awful. When my period finally comes, it is such a relief because I know it will all be over soon.

~⚬⚬~

J.,HOUSEWIFE IN HER 40's; Seattle, WA

My husband blames my moods on my period. Whenever I'm confrontational, angry, or depressed, he blames my periods. This attitude makes me furious because it is an excuse for him not to deal with any of the important issues in our marriage. Our problems are always dismissed by him as the fault of my hormones. He can never accept responsibility for even a part of our troubles. It's such a crock. Men use women's cycles as an excuse for not looking at their own problems. I'm sick and tired of being blamed for everything because I have a womb.

~⚬⚬~

S.S., SOCIAL WORKER in her 30's; Vancouver, BC

I get really sexy around the time of my periods. My husband always knows when I'm coming close to that time because I'm just so horny. It's not true that women don't want sex when they are Bleeding. I certainly enjoy it, and my husband does too. In the morning, it may look like there was a traffic accident in our bed with all the Blood everywhere, but it's worth the mess because the sex was so good.

❦

K.D., ACUPRESSURE THERAPIST in her 40's; Queen Charlotte Islands, BC

My period is a very important time of the month for me. It is a time of cleansing and rejuvenation. It is also a time when I feel closest to another world. I go very inward and connect with my centre. One of the things I have learned to do for myself at this time is not to schedule many appointments. I want my period to be a very inward, centred time. I also find I don't like to make any new decisions at this time. I always hold off until after my period before I decide something. It is also a time for me to be involved with nature a lot. I like to be out walking in the woods and by the ocean. My organs feel very open and involved with all the elements of the universe. I do less physical exercise the first couple of days of my period. I pamper myself, I love myself, I give myself that time to take care of me and say "You're O.K. You need to be loved." I give myself that mothering and fathering that I need.

❦

G.L., EXOTIC DANCER in her 20's; Los Angeles, CA

I have a very satisfying sex ritual which I like to do during my ovulation and menstrual cycle. These two times of the month are when I feel the most sexy; they also coincide with the full and new moon which adds to their power.

I begin by setting up sacred space in my room. When I do ritual, I like to really transform my space, so I use a lot of props: coloured cloths and candles for the four directions, crystals, incense, body paint, and music all help set the scene. I usually take a nice bath with herbs and bath salts before I begin. I work either skyclad or in ritual robes depending on the season.

I begin my sex magic ritual as I would any other. I call in the four quarters and invoke the Goddess and God. From that point on, I just go with the flow of my mood; I do whatever feels right and fits my purpose at the time. First of all, I want to raise and focus my energy. To do this I may drum and chant, or

I may dance to music on the stereo; anything that will put me in the proper energized mood. When I reach a certain plateau, I raise my energies further by pleasuring myself. To do this I use round polished crystals and stones. In the candlelight, listening to powerful music with my crystal on or in me, I feel so deeply in trance, it is almost unbelievable. When I Bleed the feeling is even more intense.

This type of ritual has been very healing for me. I've learned to love myself more and know that my body is a very special part of my spirituality.

⚜

V.A., OPERATING ROOM technician in her 30's; Detroit, MI

It's been ten years now since I have had a normal period. Often I will go for months at a time without one, then they will come on a few times and then stop again. The last period I had was over a year ago. My doctor says it's because I am too thin. He says I need to put on fifteen pounds and then maybe they will start up again. I keep trying to eat more but it is very difficult. I just don't want to eat and I have to force myself to eat more. One of my friends says I need to love myself more. She says I deny myself food which is the same as denying myself love. Maybe she is right, but it is so hard to feel worthy of life and love.

⚜

STARHAWK, AUTHOR AND witch; San Francisco, CA

Amenorrhea is the inability to have a period for months or years at a time. It is often connected to anorexia. I feel that cultural pressures to conform to a certain body image cause us to hate our bodies, particularly if we do not fit the stereotype of what is considered to be beautiful. Doing ritual, to affirm menstruation, will help in the healing process. Becoming comfortable with our bodies and our womanness has much to do with the cure of this.

⚜

M.E., BIOENERGETIC therapist in her late 30s; Victoria, BC

I don't think there is any work that women can do with their bodies that wouldn't get into the negative feelings we have about our bodies. Inevitably bioenergetics brings that up when people have to take a look at how they feel about their bodies. Most of us start out by thinking our bodies don't exist.

This is a very common pattern for women; not to be aware of the very subtle and continuous sensations that come from our bodies every single moment of every single day. This is a difficult area to work on because we feel so alienated; we've taken on outside opinions about our bodies, our sexuality, and menstruation for example. I don't know many women who don't feel that it's something to be embarrassed about or hidden.

⊚⟨⟩⟨⟩

E.B., EXECUTIVE SECRETARY; Chicago, IL

I have bad cramps during my periods. I feel like staying at home and relaxing at those times, but usually I can't. I have a very demanding job which won't allow me such a luxury. I wish I knew some pill or magical cure that would allow me to go on, business as usual. I've been considering having a hysterectomy for that reason, but I'm not totally sure because someday I might want to settle down and raise a family. So what to do? I'm not sure.

⊚⟨⟩⟨⟩

B.W., TEACHER IN HER 40's; Vancouver Island, BC.

At this point in my life (forty-four) the pre-menstrual period seems to last much longer than when I was younger ... from two to eight days. If it is long, then I really begin to suffer with migraine headaches and I feel like I'll explode. I feel exhausted but can't sleep, as my heart beats energetically and my mind races. Sometimes I will lie awake all night. I will have very creative ideas and come up with insights, ideas for musical compositions (I am a composer), and solutions in my day to day life.

⊚⟨⟩⟨⟩

H.S., PSYCHOLOGIST in her 30's; Los Angeles, CA

As I have gotten older, I've developed intense sensations on the first night of my flow. For one year it was so intense that combinations of yoga, breathing, self-pleasuring, love-making, marijuana, liquor, hot baths and hot water bottles, and chanting were insufficient to decrease the pain enough to allow sleep. I finally gave up and accepted a once-a-month all-nighter where I stay awake and draw, chant, self-massage, etc. Invariably the sensations lessen as the sun rises, and then I sleep.

***

M., HOUSEWIFE IN HER 40's; London, England

I was brought up with the teaching that one's period was a curse. I had severe cramps for the first twenty-four hours and heavy bleeding, so I had to stay put or I would soak.

***

M.I., COMPUTER PROGRAMMER in her 40's; Edmonton, Alta.

A healthy thirty-year-old woman I know has been suffering severe cramps since her tubal ligation. When she talked to her physician about this, she was told that it was quite common. She wasn't told of this before surgery. I had a tubal ligation ten years ago, and have experienced no problems, but I wasn't warned either.

***

E.M., STUDENT IN HER 20's; Vancouver, BC

My girlfriend used to have bad cramps, as I do. She told me that after she had her uterus dilated by a D&C, the cramping stopped. Her doctor said some women have a small cervix and when they menstruate, the pressure builds up as the Blood tries to get out, hence the cramps. After that, I remembered my mother telling me she had bad cramps until she had me, then they stopped. Well, having a child right now is not what I want to do with my life, and having a D&C doesn't thrill me either. I read in the book *Our Bodies, Ourselves* that there is this kind of seaweed that a doctor can insert that will naturally dilate the cervix. I plan to check into this to see if that may solve my problem.

***

S.T., STUDENT IN HER 20's; Portland OR

I cramp sometimes, but not a lot. I look upon this pain as a preparation for childbirth someday, so I endure the pain and flow with it. It makes me feel strong, like the Mother Earth.

∞

C.C.L., COMPUTER PROGRAMMER; Calgary, AB

I cramp a lot when I Bleed. I guess it is because I feel sad then. It's hard to let go, because I have tried for so long to get pregnant. When my period comes, I feel bad because, once again, the egg has died, the uterus is empty.

∞

K., 20'S; ONTARIO

I have never taken any drugs for menstrual pain because it is important to me that I understand the pain instead of numbing it, and I have had unforgettable experiences because I paid attention.

My first period started when I was fifteen and I don't remember any pain until I was eighteen. At that point, I began living with a man. I mention this because at twenty-two, I fell in love and moved in with a wonderful woman and, since then, I have had mild menstrual pain, if any. One time the pain was more intense than usual. I felt if I took drugs, I would not be able to respect myself as strong, and I felt that I'd be insulting my body's integrity and the integrity of my womanhood. I do make use of as many herbs as I need because herbs work with me. I can integrate them and relate to them, unlike other kinds of relief like Motrin or Pamprin.

∞

T., NURSE IN HER 40'S; Victoria, BC

One year, I had an unusually heavy flow during the time I was menstruating – or so I thought. After days of this, and an unusual smell and consistency, I went to the doctor who said I was hemorrhaging in my uterus. Though sometimes a D&C (dilation and curettage) is recommended, the less traumatic course of action is to rest, keep your feet up, and let it run its course. The doctor said that ten per cent of women get unexplained uterine hemorrhages as adults and that it often reoccurs with these same women, but that it passes on its own without interfering treatment. To rest was the obvious course of action for me. It caused no pain only tiredness, and some dizziness if I got up too quickly.

⚬⟿⟦⟧

J.N., MUSIC TEACHER in her late 40's; Victoria, BC

I feel I have been lucky not to have suffered from cramps and a lot of pain or heavy Bleeding. Recently, however, I have experienced migraines at the start and end of my period. This has gotten worse in the last two years. Usually migraines are caused by dietary problems with me, but I understand migraines are also part of the menopausal process. I think it is similar to adolescence; the hormones aren't settled down and things are changing.

I told my doctor about the migraines and he gave me a prescription. I never take anything without researching all possible side effects. Since these pills had caffeine in them, and I react very strongly to caffeine, I wasn't able to use the prescription and haven't found anything useful to help relieve the pain.

⚬⟿⟦⟧

B.E., WITCH IN HER 40's; Seattle, WA

All through my teens and early twenties I used to hate having my periods. Every month I dreaded its coming. I wasn't always regular and, when it came, it seemed always to be at the most inconvenient times. I cramped a lot and occasionally had awful headaches too. All in all, I guess I hated being a woman. It seemed to me men had it so much better than we women did. It just wasn't fair. If they had a sex change operation for women, I'm sure I'd have been the first in line.

Recently, I learned about Wicca and the religion of the Goddess. It's like I've been waiting for this all my life. Now I'm proud to be a woman. Gone are my monthly fights with my body and my Blood. I feel happier and healthier – no more headaches and almost no cramps. If someone told me ten years ago that how I felt about being a woman would affect menstrual cramps I would have laughed in their face. Now I know from personal experience that it's true.

JEAN MOUNTAINGROVE, teacher in her 50's; rural Oregon

I felt my gut cramp like a clenched fist.

In my imagination I saw an Indian, walking alone in a meadow near a stream, pausing to look up towards the mountain. I know that my mind has merged with hers.

An ancient message, reaching me like a thin scent of smoke, makes my nostrils widen in alert attention. The call is primitive, across ages: I am transfixed. Then, slowly, I sink to the Earth, my Mother, and Bleed, return my Blood to her in humble obedience.

The imperious clench in my belly reminds me that I am not a free being in command of my body. Only for a time can I choose my actions. When this internal call comes I cannot deny its claim. I can resist, with resulting pain, but I cannot stop it. When the tides rise, flooding me with inner sensation, I must focus there, withdrawing from the world.

Over the following days, returning calls were less insistent – a sharp or dull clenching like fingers around my gut with a quick or slow release. Always I was stopped by this reminder that soon I must give way. At last the flow. The heaviness and congestion breaking into dull pain and my becoming dullness. Now, such little strength, moving so slowly, resting so much, spent so soon. If I could really rest ... turn this small strength on the inwardness I am living.

Instead, I hold brittle barriers shakily in place and too often walk over fragments shattered from letting them slip.

This is my shame: I Bleed. I hide this shame with whispers and bravado, living with fear that my sluggish fingers will falter, the barriers slip to reveal my original sin, my inadequacy, my inner cavity, my nothingness.

I Bleed. I soil my bed, my clothes, my thighs. I defile myself. I must be on guard not to soil you.

I am weak. I cry at your uncaring, at your brusqueness, at your pushing energy. I hate myself, but only weakly, for there is no energy for fury.

I want to turn my face to the wall, curl up in unconsciousness, wait numbly through the interminable draining of beauty, force, and mind. My body clenches in helpless pain; mild or sharp, I can't govern it. It has its way with me.

I submit to my existence as creature, or rebel, and stubbornly drug my body and mind into ignorance of where I am, pretending to myself that nothing extra is being required of me: still I am an average person, usual. No event is shaking me into touch with millions of years of biology. The impulses in my labyrinthine interior are not to be heeded, their directions are not to be followed. No! That is just pain, not a call.

Yet, if I were to listen to the forbidden, shameful movement in my cavity what would I hear? What could I learn from such nothingness?

No! The voices of this culture are loud and insistent. "'Nothing of importance is happening ... a little inconvenience – unmentionable except to physician or druggist. If you feel anything you are neurotic. Of course if you do fall apart we will overlook it – now and then – but we can't put up with much of this immaturity from you if you expect us to ever take you even a little bit seriously."

Too long I have denied myself, turned to my wall, and numbed my awareness. Now I will choose to take myself seriously.

I will listen.

I will try to understand the messages.

I will follow them.

I have heard a call across a million years. I will answer it.

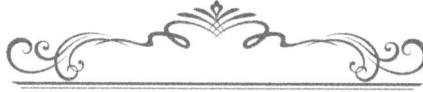

Of Bleeding and Healing

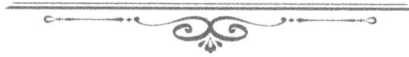

Holistic Techniques

LIKE GRASSES SWAYING in the wind
   may I be in harmony
   like a tree reaching for the sunlight
   may I be in harmony
   like water flowing over rocks
   may I be in harmony
   like the rhythmic cycles of my Blood
   may I be in harmony
   May I always be in harmony with all life
   May the Earth be my teacher and my medicine forever.
   C.W.

UP UNTIL QUITE RECENTLY, women's health issues such as menstrual problems, child bearing, and menopausal complaints were not considered to be worthy of interest or concern by the male medical profession. This lack of interest had a lot to do with the low status women often held in their societies. This isolation did have its advantages.

In the past, women's medicine, as practiced by women healers, had a far different philosophy and treatment approach than did the medicine practices of men. Historically, women's medicine was what we would today call a holistic approach towards health care. Prevention of disease was considered more important than curing disease after it had occurred. When treating a disorder, the treatment employed would be designed to treat the person as a whole being; the emotional and spiritual aspects of a condition would be considered as well as its physical symptoms to ensure a complete cure of the disease. This meant that a woman healer had to develop and become skilled in a wide variety of disciplines including herbal medicine, diet, nutrition, massage, midwifery, spellcraft, dream interpretation, and ritual magic.

Throughout the eons of time this was the hidden tradition passed down from mother to daughter. It was a simple tradition that respected life and was in harmony with the living Earth. It was also a tradition largely ignored by men until recent times.

With the rise of industrial civilizations around the world, these ancient traditions have been lost to most women. The chain has been broken and now most women no longer possess that simple earthy knowledge of how to heal themselves. They rely instead on doctors (usually men coming from a male medical tradition) to do that for them. As male doctors took over the midwife's role and began to study gynecology, the focus of women's health shifted from a holistic, preventative approach to a consideration of women's normal biological functions as disease states. No longer was childbirth, for example, viewed as a normal, natural female condition which could be dealt with easily in the security of a woman's own home. Nowadays, childbirth is treated more like a terrible disease, requiring the hospitalization of both mother and child.

Traditionally, men's medicine focuses on treating the body as a disease state. A person with a particular symptom is diagnosed and treated by drug therapy, or by surgically removing the dysfunctional part. With this methodology, it's too easy to treat the individual, not as a whole human being, but as a piece of meat for study or dissection.

For women this has meant a rise in unnecessary hysterectomies and caesarean sections at childbirth, as well as the treatment of emotional problems with dangerous habit-forming drugs.

Fortunately the picture is not totally black because that ancient holistic knowledge is not completely lost. Today both men and women healers are reviving and adding to these ancient teachings. Herbal medicine, nutrition, massage, acupuncture, peer counselling, and shamanistic ritual are being introduced as alternatives to the medical profession as equally valid forms of health care for many conditions.

In this chapter, women with knowledge in a variety of alternative health fields speak about their work and experiences. These pages are meant to make the reader aware of other alternatives. They are not meant to suggest treatment for any condition requiring professional help.

These personal stories suggest holistic healing of the self and, in turn, of the planet, Herself.

INTERVIEW WITH HERBALIST, Rosemary Gladstar; California

Herbs have been used for thousands of years in helping to heal many problems associated with menstruation. I recommend that women's gynecological problems are an area that women should treat solely on their own, or with a holistic practitioner. I very rarely recommend using orthodox medicine, as herbs tend to work best as a primary method. This is because reproductive organs are highly emotional and are the centre of life and vitality within our bodies. Herbs and holistic medicine (whole things) also vibrate with life. Consequently, these work together much better than trying to take a dead substance and kill things in our bodies.

It is interesting to note that over the centuries people have used herbs for a variety of medicinal purposes. In particular, there is a huge repertoire of herbs that are specific to gynecological problems. Most of the herbs used are common today. Frequently used herbs include ginseng, donquay, and ginger. Chaspberry is an herb that is well known in the European and Mediterranean countries. It grows in the Mediterranean and was only brought to this country within the last ten years. It has gained a wonderful reputation for helping with any kind of reproductive problem where congestion within the organs is found. Another popular herb used a lot for balancing female hormones is wild yam.

When working on the reproductive system, no matter what the problem is, I often start with the liver. This is because many hormonal problems appear to be related to the liver. Thus, cleansing and unclogging this organ helps a great deal in clearing up problems with menstruation. This makes sense because the liver not only rules the condition of the blood in our body, but also the digestion of food, and it is also a strong producer of hormones. I base my methods more on Chinese medicine, where the liver is often associated with the reproductive organs. This approach is different from Western herbology in that here, in the USA, most practitioners will recommend herbs that specifically relate to the reproductive system.

Another area I focus on is primary health. Most of the reproductive imbalances that are chronic stem from systematic ill health. Consequently, these organs aren't able to function properly. Herbs used to balance the system include nourishing plants like nettle or raspberry leaf. Watercress and oat straw are also popular. Magnesium and other herbs high in calcium are excellent for the reproductive system.

The balanced herbal formula I recommend is good food, lots of exercise, and life-style changes – which tends to be the most difficult part. However, I feel very strongly that, although making some small changes in one's approach to health is good, old habits will continue to be a problem unless some major changes are made and kept.

The herbs used are generally made into tea and given to the woman to drink for three to four months. A traditional female toner includes a mixture of strawberry leaf, raspberry leaf, oat straw, horsetail, comfrey, nettle, red clover, and something spicy, like spearmint or peppermint, for good taste. The root and bark blend tends to be stronger than most and is favoured as a foundation formula. It helps to build the liver, but is also good for the reproductive organs and helps feed the whole system.

After a foundation formula has been used for a period of time, the specific problem is looked at. If cramping is the problem, the herbs used include cramp bark and ginger, or skullcap and lobelia. A favourite blend is pennyroyal, yarrow, and catnip. Pennyroyal grows in the mountains and is excellent for relieving menstrual and pelvic cramping. It works because it brings blood to the pelvis, thus relaxing the cramps. However, it must be used properly or it can cause serious damage. Mugwort is also a favourite, not only for relieving cramps, but also for regulating cycles. Mugwort tincture has been thought to be very helpful for menstrual cramps, but it is also good for treating the absence of Bleeding.

Pennyroyal has often been used for abortions although in order for it to be effective, one must drink a large amount of it and exclude food. Many women use pennyroyal and cohoshes as a method for birth control, but technically they are abortificants. Throughout the literature on birth control, there has not been found an appropriate method using herbs. Any of the in-depth studies from various tribes on methods of birth control state that the herbs in question usually cause complete infertility or sterility.

Horsetail can be used as a tincture or made into tea. Horsetail tea is one of the best ways for replenishing calcium in the body, much better than through dairy products. It can also be used for other bodily problems, including relief from arthritis and vaginal infections.

⊙≫≪

C.H., WITCH

Three to seven days before menstruation, alternate days of luxury and self-pampering with days of exercise. For example:

day 7, mineral and bubble bath

day 6, swimming

day 5, mineral and bubble bath

day 4, jog, walk or ride a bicycle

day 3, relax with good reading material

During menses and 1 to 3 days before onset, alternate family and friend get-togethers, potlucks, spiritual rituals, and anything that is fun and stimulating with exercise.

This is an excellent treatment for PMS, headache, cramps, depression – everything that comes with menstruation. The mineral bath restores electrolyte balance. The bubble bath just smells exotic and makes us feel good. The warm/hot bath relaxes tired muscles. Exercise gets rid of prostaglandin naturally and promotes a more regulated evacuation of the uterus. Exercise also stifles water-weight gain. Being surrounded by family and friends takes our mind off minor discomforts and helps us to focus on the joy of living.

⊙≫≪

L., POET IN HER 40'S; Houston, TX

When I first started having my periods it was really painful for me. I used to have to stay in bed for two or three days. As I grew older I got so I'd try to ignore the pain, go to work anyway, and just sleep lots when I was at home. Then in 1983 I took a course in homeopathy. My teacher recommended a constitutional remedy of sulphur that really improved my periods. I had about half the pain as I'd had before. Then later in homeopathy I used siepia which is also good for your period and helped me as well.

In the last two years I've started using herbs more for my periods. I use raspberry leaves and Golden Seal tea. I figure out what herbs I should take by using a pendulum so I can't always tell you objectively why they help. I can usually tell when my periods are about to start. Then I make the tea and drink it two to three times a day for a couple days and that seems to work well for me. In the last six months I've had no cramps at all.

When I have my periods, I often have mood swings. I'll either be really hyper, or really down, and I take Bach flower essence remedies for that. They seem to be really good for balancing out my moods at that time.

B.E., WITCH IN HER 30's; rural New Mexico

For health and magical reasons, I make and use a lot of moon and sun teas. I make these teas by placing the herbs I desire in a glass jar of cold water to stand outside in the light for a prescribed period of time. Sun teas are stimulating and very quick; three to four hours in the hot sun and you have a wonderful refreshing summer drink. Some of my favorite sun teas are sage, mint, sorrel, comfrey, and borage. The moon teas I prepare in a similar manner as sun teas, but they have a deeper, more ritualistic meaning for me. I allow them to stand in the jar over one night in the moonlight. By allowing the herbs to seep slowly in the light of the sun and the moon, the tea absorbs not only the healing properties of the herbs, but it also is empowered by the light from the heavens above.

Connected to their beneficial physical properties, herbs have affects on our emotions as well. To give an example, if I am working on a particular problem like uncomfortable periods, I would choose herbs in this manner for a moon tea. I would consider my feelings first and try to choose herbs to enhance or change my mood. For cramps I would place in my jar soothing, healing herbs like comfrey, horsetail, catnip, nettle, and perhaps a little marijuana, blue cohosh, or scullcap – muscle relaxants for the pain. I might also add clear thinking herbs or borage for the courage to look within myself and see what is out of balance in my life that might be the underlying cause of the trouble.

The phases of the moon are important as well. New to full is best for invoking, the waning moon is best for banishing and the quiet introspection of the crone. If we can accept that our lives are intertwined with the natural elements and all living things, then we begin to understand how we can be influenced by all the things around us.

When I make my teas I do a ritual as I prepare them. I chant and pray, breathe, and focus my intent into them. Then I set them under the sky and invite the spirits of the sky, sun, moon, and stars to come and bless my drink. I always offer something of mine in return for the gift – some hair, my Blood, a special song. In some way I want to say thank you for the gift I will receive. Later, when I arise from my dreams to drink my moon teas with the dawn light, I feel so blessed and in harmony with the world. It is very powerful healing magic.

❦

CORNWOMAN

Let me tell you a story about how I made a special medicine for myself. For months prior to the time of the story I had been under a lot of stress. My neck and shoulders were tight all the time, and when my Bloods came, it was quite intense. I didn't want to go to the doctor and take drugs. I wanted to use herbs, but the herbs I had tried weren't quite right. I had been attracted to a highly dangerous plant which I won't name because it can be quite fatal if used improperly. The name isn't important; what I want to explain is the process. I was attracted in spite of warnings. I felt a strange kinship. Many people are afraid of this herb, but in the ancient times it was widely used as a medicine.

On a walk one day, I took a leaf of this plant, offering some of my hair as a gift. I kept the leaf a long time, holding it in my daily meditations, trying to feel the essence of this powerful plant. I prayed, dreamed, waited, and finally, one day in late summer as the moon waned (for this is a plant that belonged to Hecate), I knew it was time to collect it. A friend had told me that some of the plant I sought grew near the ocean, so my son Jes and I made a day of it at the beach. Along with our lunch I took a glass jar and a pint of vodka (not to drink but to make a tincture of my plant).

It was a warm, sunny day. We took our time strolling along the beach. While Jes played in the surf, I searched the shore for my weed. I could feel Hecate's presence drawing me; but I couldn't feel the actual plant. As the afternoon advanced I began to doubt myself. We had walked about two miles from our starting point and it was getting late. Now I realized I had to wait until the sun was just right in the western sky. The late afternoon and evening are my special times of power and it was just at that time I found a large cluster of the honoured plants I sought. While Jes played, I sang to the plants and offered them pieces of my hair. (If I had been Bleeding, I would have offered them Blood as well.) I wanted only some seeds so I broke them off and put them in my jar. When it was full, I covered the seeds with the vodka to the top of the jar and placed the lid on tight. I held the jar up to the wind and sun admiring the light on the green seeds. I sang and asked the sun and the wind to bless my medicine with their power. I felt a strong pull to bathe the jar in the sea so I walked out into the water and immersed the jar in the waves. I felt good, strong, and directed by my power to do each step. As I sat once more upon the beach I noticed a beautiful green stone near my feet. It was unique among the grey and black rocks around it. Its colour was like my seeds. I picked it up and placed it on the jar, taking it with me when we left. I wanted to keep it near the jar as the medicine grew in power.

That night I placed the jar and the stone in the moonlight. I left them in sun and moon for three days and then placed them in my darkened herb cupboard to finish working.

Though I know I must be careful and treat this plant medicine with respect, when I've used it, the herb has been kind. I'm glad I have it, though I seldom use it because it is so powerful. What I want to share is the process of how this medicine was made. If we are quiet and centred in our body and in our wombs, the plants will speak to us. We can know what herb will help us and where and how to get it. The wisdom in books is a good beginning, but it is only that. The wisdom we can tap into when we look within is the true wisdom.

When deciding what herbs to use, trust your instincts. Herbs react differently with different people so always use ones with which you have an affinity. Using herbs isn't the same as using drugs, though drugs are often made from herbs. Herbs have a soul and they have feelings. They can give you their power, but they must be approached with love and thankfulness to receive all their blessings.

❦

INTERVIEW WITH PATRICE Haan, herbalist; Victoria, BC

Probably my favourite herb for women's concerns is red raspberry leaves. Part of that stems from the fact that they grow in my garden so they are readily available to me all year round, but red raspberry is a wonderful tonic for the female reproductive organs. It's a nice blood cleanser, slightly calming, and it tones up the glandular system of the body. Specifically it is a uterine tonic when women are Bleeding, pregnant, or in labour. A lot of their energy is centred in that area. It is a good herb to have around. There are a lot of wonderful stories and supportive case histories to show how this herb has helped women through difficult pregnancies and deliveries.

Whenever I am talking to a woman about her menstrual cycle, I ask about what she is eating. I spend time with her focusing on what foods other than herbs she will be taking into her body. Given the nature of her diet, I might also suggest other herbs to help cleanse and/or build up her whole body. For example, if a woman is under a lot of stress, drinking a lot of coffee, and eating a lot of processed foods and sugar, I might suggest she first take dandelion root to help cleanse the liver and then use herbs that will directly focus on the female organ system.

My own personal experience has been with dysmenorrhea. I used to have really painful cramping that would lay me low for a few days each month. Fortunately, I've managed to come up with a couple of remedies that suit me quite well. I've tried them on other women who have also used them with success.

The first remedy is eating lots of alfalfa and dark leafy green vegetables like kale, broccoli, or spinach. You can take alfalfa either in tablets or drink it in tea. Alfalfa is a blood cleanser which is useful in an all-round way, but specifically, if the blood is freed of toxins, it tends to clot less and flow more evenly. Alfalfa also provides lots of vitamins and minerals which help the system. Calcium is one of the most important of these because it relaxes the muscles which will help with cramping. Alfalfa and raspberry make a very good blend of uterine tea.

My actual cramp relief formula is based on a formula used by my teacher, Michael Tierra. It is a combination of cramp bark, squawvine, and angelica or donquai. Donquai is the Chinese version of the plant and is the most balanced, but the angelica that grows in this country is equally good. This formula is very tonifying to the whole reproductive system. It either stops the cramping entirely, or at least makes it bearable so that you can function.

I make this formula into a tincture rather than a tea because it is easier to carry a little bottle with me in my purse. I can use it as often as needed, as much as an eye dropper full every hour or so on particularly bad days. Quite simply, a tincture is made by allowing the herbs to soak in vodka for about two weeks. Then the liquid is strained through a cloth and bottled for use. Tinctures are more concentrated than teas so you need only take a few drops to get excellent results. One of the other things I like about this cramp formula is that it uses plants indigenous to this continent. These plants were used by the American Indians. Both cramp bark and squawvine are traditional Native remedies.

In keeping with the subject of cramping, some other herbs I would suggest trying are skullcap or valerian. Black and blue cohosh skullcap are really nice herbs to help you calm down and relax when you are under a lot of stress. Black and blue cohosh are also very useful herbs both as tonics and as a relief from cramping. Valerian, for those who can tolerate it, is another good sedative and nerve relaxer. I don't suggest it as a regular treatment unless treated with respect because it is a very powerful herb.

The other herb I've used to some extent in treating the reproductive system is false unicorn root. Its primary use is as a regulator and fertility inducer. It's said in the herbal literature that if you don't want to get pregnant, don't use false unicorn root. If you want to have an absolutely beautiful reproductive system, use it, but be careful. Nettle is also a good regulator. Along with red clover it makes a good nourishing tea. Motherwort is another herb noted for its healthful effect on the reproductive system. Camomile is also really nice as a regulator and calming agent. For me, having camomile footbaths is very restorative and calming. I know one woman who uses camomile as a poultice right on her belly over her womb when she has cramps and reports it works well.

⟋⟍⟋⟍⟋

INTERVIEW WITH COLLETTE Gardener on herbal remedies; rural Oregon

Since I work with herbs, many women ask me about herbs to help with problems with their menstrual periods, such as cramping and PMS. It's good to take a supportive role when dealing with moon cycle problems. A quick self-analysis can be very helpful – herstory of cycles, types of birth control used, surgeries or infections involving the pelvic area-all are important factors. Also, it's good to look at your body type. If you are thin and small-boned and cold, warming, supportive herbs might work well. If you are solid, big-boned, with a slow metabolism, an herb that is stimulating or an energy mover might be right for you.

When choosing an herb, it's good to make a list of all the things that it does – diuretic, mineral-rich – any of its characteristics – warming, cooling, nutritive, etc. Use your imagination. Much of this is intuitive – how does the herb feel to you, which herb fits you best? Are there contra-indications? Is it safe for long-term use? Research as much as possible before picking an herb to use.

One of the key factors in having a healthy menstrual cycle is adequate nutrition. Herbs can be very helpful here as many of them are very high in vital nutrients as well as having actions that relieve uncomfortable symptoms. They get to the root of the matter as well as dealing with the other problem.

Many women have problems with cramps which can be caused by many things. By increasing their calcium intake a week to a week-and-a-half before

Bleeding starts, some women are helped. Sometimes water retention and premenstrual achy feelings are also relieved by increased calcium intake. In the latter half of our menstrual cycle, the need for calcium increases. Our body can respond to this sudden loss by releasing stress-related hormones, causing cramps, water retention, and pooling of Blood in the centre of the body.

Many herbs are high in calcium; for example, alfalfa, red clover, nettles, oat straw, wild oats, and horsetail in small amounts. Alfalfa, red clover, nettles, and horsetail are also slightly diuretic to help rid the body of excess water. Nettles are very supportive of the kidneys, and red clover and alfalfa are excellent blood and liver cleansers, and this is helpful in the last half of the cycle when the liver is working at full capacity to break down the hormones created during the cycle. This is one of the great things about herbs – they work on many levels to help restore balance.

Sometimes women are getting adequate minerals in their diet, but they aren't absorbing them well. One way to deal with this is to take a small amount of tea or tincture that is bitter fifteen to thirty minutes before meals. Swish it around in your mouth before you swallow. This stimulates the salivary glands in your mouth and the enzymes and acids in the stomach that help break down your food.

Digestive bitters will also help stimulate bile production which plays an important role in helping us absorb the vitamins and minerals in our food. They can help relieve gas as well. Some examples of good herbs are Roman camomile, catnip, and yellow dock. Wormwood and rue have also been traditionally used, although they are now considered safe for internal use by the FDA.

There also seems to be a correlation between getting enough essential fatty acids and proper hormone function. Essential fatty acids are naturally occurring raw oils like those found in nuts and avocados. Most of our oil intake is refined, saturated, cooked, or hydrogenated. Cutting back on these eases the burden on our liver and other organs, and makes room in our diet for foods containing essential fatty acids.

In terms of the pain of cramps, there are many herbs to be tried. Burdock is an excellent tonic herb that has an affinity for the pelvic area, but not as much pain relief action. It's gentle, nutritive, and cleansing to the liver and blood. The root is most commonly used although the seed is also powerful. It is warming and gently acts to unblock any stuck energy in the pelvic area. A good ally for any woman with cycle or pelvic problems. Its deep root lets us know that it goes to the root of the problem energywise. Herstorically it has been used for longstanding or deep-rooted imbalances.

For pain I recommend motherwort. It is a mild nervine, emmenagogue, and slight vasodilator that is reputed to have a tonic effect on the heart. Motherwort means mother's herb. It's a pain reliever and antispasmodic. Some women use it for ovulation pain as well as cramping. It's a gentle tonic for the pelvic area.

For women whose cramping is hot and fiery, and who are very nervous, scullcap can be useful. For some women it only calms them down without relieving the pain. Scullcap helps cool and calm the nerves. It contains vitamins and mineral-like substances that feed and nourish the nervous system.

Yarrow taken as a hot tea helps draw Blood away from the centre of the body. So it often helps with the type of cramping that comes from energy pooled and stuck there. It's also helpful for women who bleed excessively.

Pennyroyal and thyme also help bring blood away from the centre of the body, but they are slight emmenagogues, so they may increase bleeding slightly. They can be helpful when there's pelvic congestion and not much flow. Pennyroyal should never be used during pregnancy and is never taken internally as an essential oil. It can be fatal. Herstorically, it has been used as an abortificant, although it isn't always reliable, and can cause serious side effects in a pregnancy that continues.

THE MAGICAL USE OF Herbs, Collette Gardener, herbal consultant; rural Oregon

I use the herbs I gather for magic in two ways. I hang them in little pillows around my bed, or I burn them in an abalone shell or smudge pot. I find it especially helpful to do this the day before I begin my period, or on the first day or two that I am Bleeding.

One of the herbs I especially like to use in this way is blue vervain. It grows wild in dry, sunny areas and has very beautiful bluish purple flowers. From mid-June through July, the flowers can be harvested and dried for later use. Blue vervain is a nervine when taken internally; when burned, the flowers have the same property on a psychic level. The herb also provides needed protection for the psychic channels that are so open and vulnerable during menstruation. If you burn it just before you Bleed, it provides a shield around your psychic energy so you can safely open up. It seems to help to re-establish that connection we all have with the universe. It helps to restore your faith in the powers within yourself as well as with out. It's a very calming and protective herb, very grounded, yet allowing you out in the world at the same time.

Another herb I use a lot at this time is mugwort. it's a very psychic, magical herb whose properties include the opening of the third eye. It is also the bringer of dreams. In the old days, carrying a sprig of mugwort was the symbol of a healer. I burn mugwort, or tie it to my bed, or put it in a dream pillow that I place under my head when I sleep. Mugwort is a very witchy plant, sacred to the goddess Artemis. I find it very interesting that it's in the same family as the native sage that the Indian people here use.

Another herb I use is pine needles. I'll burn them when I feel exposed to some unclean energy, or to magically protect myself from germs. They are also good to take as a tea, being very resinous and disinfectant. I like them because they are easy to get as well.

A good one I use as well is sage, though I don't use it so much during my Moon time as it seems too dry for me. If something really intense has gone down, then I will burn it. I also burn angelica at my Moon time. I use the leaf as I believe it calls in angels and provides protection for your higher self. Whatever tradition you follow, it calls in the faeries or divas or angels and asks for their assistance as well as bringing out a sense of responsibility in yourself. You call on forces outside yourself when you use angelica.

Sometimes I also burn rosemary. Rosemary is very cleansing so when my brain feels a little fuzzy I burn it and it seems to perk me up and lighten the energy around me.

I use herbs magically at other times of the month, too. Just recently, I found an old recipe that combines burning hazel buds, rose petals, thyme, and pine needles. It helps you to see faeries. I'm going to try it. I also get into burning on my stove a little of what I have on my spice rack each day. Lately I've been getting into a lot of sweet spice like cloves, cinnamon, nutmeg, and pine needles. Sometimes I burn traditional incense like myrrh or copalgum, but they seem so old by the time I get them that they have lost much of their vital force. I think of such herbs as very sacred, but I only use them on celebratory occasions. I also want to acknowledge that the herbs I find around me are sacred, too, and I use them as much as possible.

INTERVIEW WITH K.J., nurse and midwife in her 40's; Portland, OR

Often women come to me for validation of their menstrual pains. Most men doctors tell them that PMS and cramping is mainly in their minds. I personally believe that the main reason women struggle with PMS and pain is because this culture tells women to ignore the pain and carry on with their lives. The same thing happens with childbirth. I tell my women to go to bed with their babies. I tell them to nurture themselves; they don't need to be cooking or cleaning or entertaining. They need to go to a quiet place and be alone. They need to allow themselves to be cared for. This culture says you are not okay if you do that; you aren't healthy and whole, but we are!

It's okay to nurture ourselves. If a woman comes to me with PMS, the first thing I try to do is get her to take time for herself. She can use me as an excuse. I've even written it out on prescription pads for women who say their husbands would never allow it. Women have had wonderful results with this treatment alone. I have a lot of rage towards this culture that denies us what is so normal.

A BIRTH STORY TOLD by K.J.

A little while back I had a client come to me who had a caesarean delivery of a six pound baby five years before. She was pregnant again and she wanted to have a vaginal birth. After a c-section this is called a v-bac. Her c-section had been done because her baby wouldn't fit through her pelvis (medically known as a CPD). At the time of the birth, her doctor hadn't been in town and she was afraid of her substitute doctor. She had laboured a long time and had dilated very slowly so they did a c-section. Most women don't get a second chance for a vaginal delivery if they had a c-section for CPD at an earlier birth.

This client was adamant that the reason she hadn't been able to deliver normally was because she hadn't known or trusted the new doctor. She said she had not been allowed to be in a position of comfort to her, but was made to lie in bed with her legs in the stirrups as the doctor wanted. She felt that if she could just squat, her pelvis would open and let the baby out.

Well, under the circumstances, having this discussion was outside the scope of my practice. I couldn't say yes to her without an agreement from my back-up physician to allow her a trial of labour. He talked to her about the risks involved and she was very willing to take the chance. Her plan was to come to the hospital late in her labour, and she did. She came in when she was seven centimetres dilated. Things went exactly perfect; her water broke spontaneously, there was thick meconium. The baby was being stressed out by her labour, but he was already sitting in the lowest point in her pelvis so that was good. There were some really scary things happening around this birth but the woman asked to squat so the nurse and her partner helped her and she squatted and pushed for an hour. She put so much effort into it that her pelvis opened and she delivered vaginally a seven and a half pound baby. This second baby was a pound and a half bigger than her first delivered by c-section because, supposedly, it wouldn't fit.

Afterwards, the rejoicing was so incredible because this woman did what couldn't be done and because she believed in herself. Even though the baby had problems and had to stay in the hospital for five days, there was such a feeling of festivity around this birth. I get high just recalling it now.

A lot of women come to me because they didn't like the birthing position in which they were forced to deliver at previous births. My feeling is that you will know instinctively the position that is comfortable for you. A lot of my clients deliver on their sides with their legs drawn up high to their chin. There's something about squatting that helps to open the pelvis. I've had women lie in bed throughout their entire labour and when it is time to push they will throw themselves out of bed to be upright so they can squat and open their pelvis.

J.Z.N., PSYCHIC READER in her 40's; Victoria, BC

I think the single most important discovery in the last little while has to do with how women accept their femininity, their womanhood, and their bodily cycle. I have found that women who grew up learning to be ashamed of being female tend to have more trouble with their cycle in general.

I don't think any woman is totally free of discomfort all the time. You may go along for a while okay, but every once in a while, because of stress or a temporary chemical imbalance, you may have a period where you wonder what is going on in there. What I do for those times is drink herb teas. Raspberry leaf is my favourite tonic for toning the uterus. I find that two cups at the onset of my period works well. I like to mix raspberry with spearmint because of the effect on the digestive system. I use camomile as well for headaches and digestive troubles around that time, too. The fresher the herbs are, the better. I also wonder about the difference between wild and cultivated herbs. I think that wild would be the more potent of the two.

For regulating women's cycles, I recommend using light. Louise Lacy has written a book called *Lunaception*. She worked with light to control and regulate the menstrual cycle. She maintains that girls are menstruating earlier now because of our constant bombardment with artificial light. I feel that light has a lot to do with the glandular system and particularly the pituitary and its regulating hormones.

To begin regulating your body's cycle, you have to first get acquainted with your body as it is, and for that I like the basal temperature method. You take your temperature either last thing at night or first thing in the morning before you get up. You need to do this method over a long period of time to see patterns because your body temperature is affected by so many things; stress, a cold, lack of sleep, or poor diet can all affect your temperature. Start by recording it on graph paper. Your temperature will be lower before ovulation and higher after ovulation when the yellow bodies are present. Louise Lacy also recommends keeping a journal. The entries don't have to be huge as long as they are regular. I think this is a very effective method of inner exploration and getting acquainted with yourself. Louise talks about how to regulate your cycle once you have explored where you are at. She talks about sleeping in a dark room for all but four days of the month when you sleep with a dim light on in your room the whole night. The light represents the light of the full moon. She maintains that in our ancient past our cycles were regulated by moonlight and hence women were quite regular. She claims that by reproducing these conditions, modern women can regulate their cycles quite effectively.

Of course the next best way to regulate yourself is by living with, or close to, other women who are regular. It never seems to fail. You will clock to it and once in a while you will all be ovulating around the same time. Of course, if you move out, you may become irregular again. However, for the short term, it is a good method.

INTERVIEW WITH KATHLEEN de Bucy, practitioner of Shiatsu and Jin Shin Do acupressure; Victoria, BC

If a woman was to come to me with a case of PMS, I would start by reviewing with her what her symptoms might be. Then I would take the pulses on the twelve meridians that run like rivers throughout the body. I would do this to see where any imbalances between the meridians might be. After checking the twelve pulses I would have a rough picture of what was going on in her body. Then, as she lay on the table, I would press with my thumb and fingers on various points along the meridians to see if they were tender. I would then hold these points with heavy or light pressure depending on whether or not the energy in that area needed to be sedated or enhanced. I would also ask the patient to help me by breathing deeply which helps to release the points as I press on them. Jin Shin Do or Shiatsu acupressure techniques aren't supposed to be painful treatments – only a pleasant discomfort of release of tension should be experienced by the patient. As the energy blocks are released a patient will feel the energy in different ways. You might feel a buzzing sensation, or it may feel like pins and needles. What I am doing is trying to get rid of energy blocks that cause discomfort or illness, and to balance the rivers of energy throughout the body. The Orientals believe in the polarity of Yin and Yang, meaning that there is a balance of positive and negative energies in our bodies which need to be in balance and in touch with the universe as a whole. What that means is, for example, that if there is a crisis in our lives and we are in balance, we can flow through it without getting blocked or stuck. If the energies of the body are out of balance, then illness or emotional stress is caused.

An acupressure treatment takes about an hour and a half. By the time it is over you should have a sense of well being. You may have pounded on the table in anger, cried in grief, or trembled in fear, but at the end there should be a sense of harmony and being in touch with the universe and your own centre.

I've noticed that the kind of treatment I do on clients who are on their periods is a very light touch, a tonifying type of treatment. Usually women are very sensitive at that time, especially on the yin meridians of liver, spleen, and kidney. They are also very emotional, so what would be considered a light treatment at other times of the month, during menstruation can bring on great emotional release.

When I am pressing acupressure points along the spleen meridian a woman can let go of excess worries because worry is associated with the imbalance of this particular area. She can let go of the worry and then feel more loving toward everybody and take time to nurture herself. I find there is a lot of imbalance in the spleen meridian in women mainly because they are mothers and give out nurturing to everybody without receiving any for themselves.

The wonderful thing about oriental medicine is that there are three aspects when a point is released; the physical, the emotional, and the spiritual energies are balanced to work together. What that means is that in the physical realm, a point may be very sore or tight. We would say it is well armoured or very yang. The emotional aspect of that would be related to the emotion associated with that particular meridian. For example, a release along the kidney meridian would bring up the emotion of fear. This could be fear of something happening today, ten years ago or in early childhood, or even in past lives. The body doesn't forget these things but holds on to them. There are layers and layers of old emotions that need to be released in all of us, no matter who we are. Then, there is the spiritual. Using the liver as an example, what also comes out when releasing the liver meridian is anger and depression. Releasing the emotions of the liver meridian, then, allows us, on a spiritual level, to become who we really are because it frees the will to act on the true spirit within. So, in a treatment, as I release these points, all aspects can come into play or only one or two aspects may be dealt with.

Out of the twelve meridians in the body, there are three that are the most important when dealing with menstruation. The kidney is connected with the water element. Its emotional aspect is fear. The second is the liver meridian and its element is wood. Its emotional aspect is anger. The third is the spleen meridian and its element is earth with the associated emotion being love, compassion, or sympathy.

With a woman, these meridians are being brought into action more so than with a man because of the monthly cycle that takes place. Often there will be an imbalance in these meridians if the woman hasn't been taking care of herself. What we need to do in this case is build up the energy in these three meridians so they are balanced out with the other meridians.

One of the problems associated with PMS is low energy. This happens because the kidney meridian is using a lot of energy to prepare for menstruation. The kidney meridian is known as the storehouse of the chi (or life force). After ovulation a lot of energy is needed to nurture the ovum and build a nest for implantation. This of course depletes the body of chi. This also puts stress on other body organ systems. The kidney meridian must be tonified so it has enough energy to reach out and energize other organs of the body as it normally does. This is why an imbalance in the kidney meridian is associated with fatigue, edema and anxiety. A good point to press here is kidney six which is called illuminating. It is located one finger below the inner ankle bone and slightly back in the notch. This point calms urogenital imbalances which helps to relieve fear and anxieties that women often experience around menstruation. As its name suggests, it will help you to see your situation more dearly.

The spleen meridian is worked on because its main function is to control the blood flow. Cramps, low back pain, headaches, and breast tenderness are all caused by stagnant blood syndrome which is caused by a spleen imbalance. What we need to do is get that energy moving again. There are two points that are very helpful. Spleen ten translated as the "blood sea is the first. To find this point straighten your leg and on the inside of the leg in the muscle, two fingers above the knee, you will find a tender point and that is spleen ten. That point is particularly wonderful for getting the energy moving throughout the meridian and is a point all women should know. Spleen six is another good point located four fingers above the ankle, on the inside of the leg, right up against the bone. You can feel this area of tenderness. This point is called the three yin crossing because all three yin meridians pass through that spot. It is an excellent point to press for any female problems because it helps direct the energy flow between all three yin meridians concerned with a woman's cycle.

The liver is the meridian the Chinese say stores the blood. It also neutralizes many poisons in our bodies like alcohol or drugs. Because of its many functions, the Chinese believe it is an important aspect of conscious and unconscious thought. It is a controller of psychological problems such as anger or depression. If a woman is depressed or very emotional around her menses there is usually a problem or imbalance with the liver meridian. When balancing out this meridian, a good point to know is liver three. It is located at the base of the webbing between the first and second toe. This point is called supreme rushing. It helps release the will so that a woman can become in control of her life and realize her creative potential.

Personally, if I find my period is a little prolonged in arriving, I do some yoga poses, as well as pressing the above-mentioned points. I find that really helps to bring on my period. The first yoga position I do is called "the bow" and it stretches the bladder meridian on the back and all the yin meridians running down the front of the body. All the yin meridians are important in menstruation. What you do is, by lying down on your stomach on the floor, you reach back, and, by bending your knees up, clasp your ankles. Then on an inhaled breath, you raise your shoulders and legs off the floor as if you were forming a circle or bow. You hold your breath, then on an exhale you return your body to the floor. I do that about five times and it really stretches the abdominal area.

The other one I do is the virasana. It stretches the stomach and spleen meridian which runs down the legs. This one is done sitting in the Japanese zazen position; your ankles on either side of your buttocks. Then you lean back so you are laying on the floor with your knees folded back on either side of your body. You stretch your arms back behind your head and exhale. You can really feel a stretch throughout your whole body. It's like a breath of fresh air happens for me when I do that. On the exhalation you release the stretch. I do this for about ten minutes.

The other one I do is the Cobra where you lie on your stomach again and put your palms to the floor in line with your shoulders. Then on the inhalation, you raise your trunk up and arch your back. Meanwhile, you keep your pelvis and legs on the floor so you get a really good stretch through the chest area. On the exhale, lower your chest to the floor again. I do this about five times. I find these poses to really help a lot. Another thing I do is self-help shiatsu. I do this on a daily basis. It takes about ten minutes and it stimulates thirty-one key acupressure points in the body. These are points on all the twelve meridians of the body that you do to yourself. The points are held with the breath in a certain procedure and I find this really cuts down on PMS for me. It also regulates my menstrual flow and gets rid of a lot of breast. soreness as well.

As for my diet during my period, I find that miso soup is good. It provides all the proteins and B vitamins I need. I also try to stay away from salads and other cold foods. I find they cool down my body which seems to make my internal contractions more severe. So the first couple of days, I like to drink soups and teas high in calcium. Horsetail, nettle, oat straw, and camomile with anise or mint for flavour is a good combination. Raspberry leaf tea is good too.

I try to dress warm during my periods. I have a special pair of red leg warmers that have nice sparkles in them. I love to put them on and know I am nurturing my yin meridians as I do.

I also do a lot of hara breathing or deep belly breathing. You inhale to the count of four and expand the belly, hold for the count of four and then as you exhale to the count of six, you contract the belly muscles back up against the spine. I will do that sometimes for a half hour or until I feel relaxed. The reason for doing hara breathing is to get me out of my head and back into my body so I can feel what is happening with my body. In the physical aspect, this breathing technique massages and revitalizes the internal organs. It also helps me to feel I am in control of emotional situations.

INTERVIEW WITH AMARRAH Joy Eboney, holistic health counsellor and dance therapist; Victoria, BC

It's interesting to me how certain types of people are drawn to certain types of healers. Women who have come to me with severe mental disorders and emotional upsets around the time of their menstruation are women who are malnourished. The first thing I would do before we even got into the emotional stuff would be to deal with nutritional problems. I would recommend a broad base support vitamin and mineral supplement. This would include extra B vitamins and glandular support substances. I've seen this combination alone bring women out of their psychological problems. Then menstruation becomes the very normal and easy process that I feel it ought to be. This has certainly been the case for my clients and myself. I see now that a lot of my previous discomforts around and during menstruation were due to a lot of vitamin deficiencies. After the physical deficiencies are cleared up, then if women want to deal with the spiritual aspects of their period, all their energy would be free to devote to that task.

To be more specific about what substances I would recommend; hypoglycemia, low adrenal function, and PMS are all related so supporting the adrenal glands is the first step in helping the situation. Many women drink coffee and eat a lot of sugar around the time of their period which increases the chances of them having difficult periods. Supporting the adrenals with supplements will, in turn, help the pancreas. The pancreas stabilizes blood sugar which affects our mood swings. Taking extra vitamin B is important. About fifty milligrams of each member of the B group will help your body cope with the mental and physical stresses of that time of the month – many women need the glandular substance as well for all the glands, because they all work together. It seems that in my work I've found that when the glands aren't in balance there comes with that a whole host of emotional problems. Thinking in the sense of yoga philosophy, the glands symbolize on the physical level what the chakras symbolize on the astral level. When the chakras are out of balance there will be the same emotional problems. Taking supplements that contain all the known vitamins and minerals, with added amounts of all B complex and glandular substance, gives your body the material it needs from a nutritional standpoint to deal with day to day living.

This gives you an idea of what you need to take. Many health food stores sell these kinds of products. If it does not work after a while it is probably not high enough in potency. We all operate at different levels of biochemistry and emotion. It is important to try different amounts until you find one that works well for you. When we start experimenting with different formulas, I use muscle testing or dousing to determine the correct amount that a person may need. This is another problem people come to me with. They have been taking certain vitamins that don't seem to be working for them. The reason is that vitamins don't work by themselves. One vitamin may need ten others to get the most out of that one. That is why I recommend a complete supplement to begin with. A woman can be on a good diet and taking some supplements and still be malnourished because you need all the vitamins and minerals known. A better formula yet would be to include various herbs along with good diet and a complete supplement. I don't know much about which particular herbs to take, but I do know that vitamins and minerals work better when there are herbs present in the body and, in tum, you get more out of taking herbs when you are also taking supplements.

A person should muscle test the herbs they want to take to see if they are the right ones. Some people are very sensitive to certain herbs, but I do recommend using them with vitamin supplements. It just seems obvious to me that if a person is starving, then feed them first. If there is emotional stuff left over then we can work on it. Most people who come to me are helped by just working on the nutritional stuff.

When you decide on a particular program, whether it be herbs, vitamins, or a combination, it is best to plan to do it for at least three months. Some people feel rejuvenated and strong within a couple weeks, but others take much longer to start feeling the changes happening in their bodies. So, if you are not prepared to do a program for at least three months either financially or psychologically, leave it a little while until you are ready. If you start a program, then, in two weeks, either don't feel better, or run out of money and get discouraged, you'll doubt that it can help you and of course, then, it won't. Wait to start a new program until you are ready to see it through to the end.

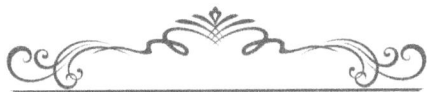

Blood of the Ancients

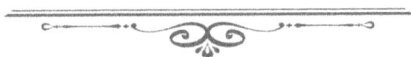

Female Shamanism, Ancient and Modern

OUR SHAMANIC ROOTS
There is a bond of Blood that binds us
linking women throughout the eons
there is a bond of Blood that binds us
it is flowing through our veins
and though the forms may pass on
there is a circle of Bleeding women
that will always remain
T.A.

IT IS MY SINCERE BELIEF that we humans have programmed into our very DNA a need for the seasonal release of energy through spiritual ecstasy. Over the years, many Native Elders I've talked to have told me that the utilization of such energies at certain times is necessary to maintain the harmony of the world. Not only Native people on this continent, but all indigenous cultures around the world, always had, and some still have, seasonal ceremonies in which group energy was directed for the healing and balance of this planet and her life forms. This perhaps is our main task today as conscious beings, helping the Earth channel this energy through our bodies and out again, focused and magnified in its healing power.

Unfortunately for our poor planet, many persons and cultures have forgotten this most ancient directive so that now we stand at the gates of destruction and don't know what to do to stop it.

On a personal level, these seasonal tides of energy can aid us in healing and spiritual growth, but here, too, most people have forgotten how to tap into and use this power. People in our world today live with a vague sense that something is missing from their lives, but they aren't sure what it is or how to find it. In such a state of unease it is no wonder that so many turn to drugs and alcohol as an escape.

Our world desperately needs a revival of meaningful seasonal spiritual ceremonies in which the ecstatic energies can be gathered and directed towards the healing of ourselves and this planet. Many of the women who have contributed writings for this chapter feel that our personal task as women is to reconnect through our bodies with the Earth Mother and work openly to defy male political power structures and help to save our world.

For this chapter, I have used a very loose definition of shamanism. I feel shamanism is a fluid term, constantly adapting to the needs of modern users. For this chapter, it refers to all healers, psychological or spiritual, who are concerned with the healing of our minds and hearts, and in aiding our spiritual growth.

୧◈◈◈

THE BLOOD MYSTERY: A Return To Our Shamanic Roots,
    Vicki Noble; Berkeley, CA

There was a time when, due to the sacred, wise Blood that spilled from us without a wound, women filled a natural role as spiritual authorities all over the "prehistoric'" world. Then, five thousand years ago, that female function was usurped by male priests and rulers, leaving a curse on women that called our Blood "unclean" and the power that came with it "demonic." All my shamanic work with women students and clients over the years has been in relation to a deep, internalized denial of female authority in all of us. In tandem with this denial in women is a projection of our disallowed spiritual authority onto men and male institutions. The current epidemic of "PMS" that debilitates so many of us each month with negative phenomena, is nothing more than a virulent symptom of this inner lack that we feel, which our culture inculcates and reinforces in us. I have unequivocally come to believe that the menstrual taboo is at the root of female oppression and subjugation.

When we Bleed each month, women experience a change of energy in what psychics call our "field." This shift in energy or power is a result of contact with the dark realm or the Dark Goddess. The Bleeding time involves access to a raw form of instinctual power that includes the ability to peer into the invisible world of the spirits and to forecast or "divine" the future. Menstrual Blood is the most potent substance on the planet in this magical sense, and in the ancient past it was used purposefully by the community. Now we disregard this extrasensory power and continue with our jobs, our home lives – "business as usual." When we behave this way, the unacknowledged "dark" power releases through us as irritation, grumpiness, headache, bloating, and other negative physical symptoms.

As a feminist, I have always struggled with this awareness. In the early days of the women's movement, I participated actively in the "women's health movement." I took part in small groups where we practised "menstrual extraction" on one another, that is, we used the plastic technology of abortion to suck out the menstrual Blood each month in five minutes, rather than having our period for several days. This seemed quite liberating at the time, as the research we were doing was aimed at removing whatever biological inequities seemed to exist between men and women so that women could be freed to govern and participate in society on an equal footing. In retrospect, I see that this was one of many misconceptions of early feminist activism, due to the lack of any spiritual base. It was impossible, then, for a "political" feminist to admit that there were significant biological differences between men and women. Now, thanks to a deepening contact with female spirituality and the Goddess, we can embrace our biological roots as the source of the politico-spiritual authority we were trying, through denial, to reclaim!

The Blood mysteries were central to the earliest shamanism. Shamanism is a form of healing that is aligned with the earth and the spiritual forces. It reveres process and does as little as possible to intervene in the natural flow of life and energy. When a shaman does intervene, it is for the purpose of harnessing the natural forces and energies at work and directing them in ways that sustain and support the process trying to happen. Images of dancing women, pregnant, wearing bird masks, or headless, adorn cave walls from 30,000 years before this era. All of their symbolism is "shamanic" and partakes of the mysterious world of the spirits and the animal powers. The early calendars from that period were notched carefully on eagle bones and they kept track of menstrual time in relation to the cycles and phases of the moon. Sculpted images of the female deity are generally painted with red ochre representing menstrual Blood, as were all the bodies our early ancestors buried in their sacred, ritual ways.

The first Blood at the altar was menstrual Blood: no wound, no death, no sacrifice. The female community almost certainly Bled together, bringing their highly-charged psychic fields into one strong, collective force for healing and regeneration of the village or tribe. (Even now girls in dormitories still synchronize around their Moon cycles!) Not only is the physical substance of menstrual Blood potent and magically effective, but the symbolic or metaphorical experience of Bleeding each month is a powerful shamanic practice. Shamans everywhere "rehearse" death during life, in order to overcome fear of it, and in order to break the barrier between life and death for the purpose of gaining access to healing power from the invisible world. A shaman "journeys" from the physical to the "spiritual" realms, from this world to the "underworld." Each journey involves a death-and-rebirth of the ego, a dissolving of ordinary consciousness, and an eventual integration of the material gained from visiting the sacred realms.

The menstrual period is a biological "Dark Moon." It is the time when the egg that did not get fertilized is shed from the womb, along with the built-up uterine lining which would have sustained a pregnancy. This is a purification or purging every month, a letting-go of what might have been but will not now ever be. Every month, adult women like snakes shed this inner skin, and emerge whole and renewed, like the lunar crescent that appears in the sky after three days of darkness. From this continual process of building up and letting go, we instinctually come to understand and accept death. In addition to this inner, innate understanding on a deep, non-rational level, there is also the presence of a dynamic force, the raw potency of the menstrual time itself. Hormonally, our yin essence (estrogen) is way down as the period approaches, and the yang substance (progesterone) is way up. There is a natural fierceness available, a volcanic energy that seems larger than the ego and even threatening to it. This is the power of the Kundalini Serpent, the awakened female force that corresponds to the "Dragon Currents" of the earth itself. When this "snake power'" erupts in us we don't know what to do with it these days because we have so few channels open to us.

What we need to do, on the simplest level, is just surrender to this force, to what the ancient Sumerians called "the law of the Great Below." The hormonal pull towards disintegration is exactly right for us, and we need to let go into the dissolution of our identities and our "normal consciousness" when the Dark Goddess calls. This means setting aside some special time and space, since otherwise we will rush around in frenetic and outer-directed ways. Brook Medicine Eagle suggests the creating of "menstrual lodges" and places where women can come to be by themselves or with other Bleeding women. In this way, we can honour the deep quiet within us and make an opportunity for the spiritual forces to speak to and through us. A sacred time-out allows for dreaming and journal-keeping, prayer, healing, and quiet renewal.

Personally, when I Bleed, I like best of all to re-enact the ancient sacred temple customs. In India, there are remnants today of the female-centred religion that included sexual initiation transmitted by a female guru in her "red" power. One of the worst oppressions of the menstrual taboo is the forbidding of sexual intercourse during a woman's period. This taboo has made women aware of our innate power and the natural tendency toward ecstasy which releases through the menstrual experience. Sexuality at this time of the month partakes of the Dark Goddess, rather than the more relationship-oriented quality of the ovulation time. There is no pro-creation urge here, no interest in caretaking, or even "love" in a personal sense. The Dark Goddess is impersonal, archetypal, and autonomous. She comes through a Bleeding woman as a force toward ecstatic creative expression. She celebrates herself through us, opening the physical senses, yet freeing something beyond that. There is an opportunity here to break from ordinary form and consciousness, for the soul to take flight through the delight and pleasure and sensate focus of the body.

My husband and I look forward to my bleeding time as our ritual time – the most sacred, enriching, unifying time of our marriage. Without a celebration at this time, something gets out of balance between us. It is a time when he has learned, over the years, to surrender to this tremendous force of the Dark Goddess, to honour and cherish its aggressive movements, its insatiable and unquenchable fire. It is indeed demanding, and he and I have both had to learn that the demand is not a personal one. It is not coming from me, but from a deeper, less personal place within me. The great serpent force demands satisfaction and creative expression. She comes through me during this auspicious time as electrical voltage and fiery power that loves to be channeled into passion and tantric bliss. It is healing for us both, and, if we take seriously the tantric scriptures, it no doubt heals our family and community as well.

In North American Native culture, the word "wakan" means sacred. It is often translated as the Great Spirit, seemingly male, who created the world and enspirits it. But Wakan Tanka is the White Buffalo Woman who came to bring peace to the world; and the word "wakan" also means "menstrual." What was originally "wakan" on this planet has been demonized and made filthy, and it is up to women today to reclaim the sacred quality of female source energy from this false definition. Ultimately, women will have to do this by Bleeding together once more, to contact again the magical powers and abilities we once had as a group. In the meantime, each one of us can bring her Bleeding time back into the temple. Each month, if each woman will simply respect and love her Blood, feed it to her plants, and anoint her candles with it, offer it to the Mother at her altar, share it with a lover, or revel in it herself, then consciousness will begin to follow this activity, catalyzing a deep, transformative healing process. The sleeping serpent Kundalini, once aroused, can't be stopped from going on her undulating path to liberation.

SACRED TIME, SACRED Way,
Brook Medicine Eagle; Helena, MT
Too many people-both men and women-have forgotten to honour the time of women's Blood. Much is suffered from incomplete knowledge of this Blood and its meaning. The time has come for us to awaken and again find

the depth of meaning that Mother Earth and Father Spirit gave us through it.

Through our adoption of European puritanical ethics, and through our human forgetfulness, we have ceased acknowledging the deep significance of women's wombs and their Blood – which make possible the creation of the human race. Many see women's Blood as bad, negative, or unclean and feel that women should hide themselves and be ashamed during this special time. Even some who understand differently create this feeling in the way they handle women on their Moon time around ceremonies and special functions; women are quite often asked to leave the circle without adequate explanation of the reasons. Thus the women feel banished and unclean.

This has come about as male medicine teachers and sweatlodge leaders have come out among the people without their female counterparts. In the tribes with which I am familiar, the medicine man did not formerly act alone or have to handle everything; with him was his wife or female helper, always there to help him and to handle any issues relating to women. Many who lead ceremonies today either do not have the knowledge or the time to instruct women who come on their Moon time. Yet this is something that must be done so learning can take place, and the dishonouring end.

The time has come for anyone who does ceremony and excludes women to take responsibility for honouring those on their Moon time before they leave the group, by giving them adequate guidelines on how their energy can best be used, and by reminding them of the great power of this experience they are having. Since Moon time is the most receptive of the whole two-legged experience, women can be instructed simply to find a peaceful place nearby, go into quiet meditation, look through the now transparent veil into the Great Mystery, and call forth vision for themselves and their people. A special time can be set aside after the ceremony for these women to bring back to the community whatever thoughts, intuitions, visions, or dreams have come to them as they sat apart. In this way, even as they sit apart, the women sit in an honoured place. Something this simple would completely change the complexion of Moon-time women's experience around ceremonial functions, and would benefit everyone.

It can also be explained to all present, that because the feminine comes first in all things, and thus holds great power, much energy is whirling about each woman in her most feminine time, whether or not she can perceive and guide it. Just as with all our energy, this whirling energy affects everything and everyone around, but in a more profound way because of its great power. Thus it can indeed change the direction or movement of a ceremony. As we all become more sensitive to subtler energies, we will have a deeper understanding within ourselves of how this energy affects events and people, and how best to use it and ourselves during this time. If we perceive it ourselves, then no one has to tell us what is happening-we will know very deeply ourselves.

There is a sacred rite among the Lakota people given them in vision to Slow Buffalo by White Buffalo Calf Pipe Woman a long time ago. In his vision, Slow Buffalo saw a great people bringing a girl child to a sacred centre place, a buffalo wallow. These people all turned into buffalo, and the girl into a buffalo calf; a large bull came and purified this calf with red powder, then all came and licked her. He understood this to mean that this young one would then go forth and bear fruit in a sacred manner, travelling to the end of the four ages. She would teach her children, too, to walk the path of life in a sacred manner.

This rite is performed when a young girl becomes a woman, when her first Moon-time Blood appears. The purpose of the rite is to purify her, honour her, and help her to realize that the change taking place in her is a sacred thing, that she will now become Mother and be able to bear children. Among the Lakota people, after the rite is performed, all people come and touch the young woman, for now she has holy power.

Several years ago, a vision came to me which I am just beginning to understand. It seems connected to this honouring that is awakening again in our young women. I looked into the future and saw a buffalo cow standing facing me. Near her head was an oblong white object several feet long which she began to lick. At first the object seemed to be a natural salt rock. It became like a newborn white calf which the cow licked into aliveness. The baby eventually rose to her feet and suckled, full of life. What I saw represents to me the rebirth of something sacred, re-awakening to the specialness of the feminine and women's Moon-time Blood. We serve, as adults, to bring these ways to life once more.

It is important that we begin to honour the first Blood and visions of our young women. The Lakota rite, called *Her Alone They Sing Over*, is very beautiful and contains the important elements of purification, honour, and realization of the sacred. Certainly not all who read this are Lakota or red people, yet other cultures all over the world practice similar ceremonies. All of us must awaken to the urgency of these kinds of rites for the honouring and instruction of our young women. More spiritual education and honouring of this special gift of creation might help young women cherish this gift and not squander their capacity for creation unwisely and prematurely.

Now I ask you to reawaken your own traditions in some way, to create the basic elements of such a rite of passage for your daughters. Call upon White Buffalo Woman. It is time.

THE WOMEN'S LODGE,
Guaba Guarikgku; Pitsburgh, PA

As far back as can be traced, the power of creating new life has been the source of ritual magic. The very fact that women Bleed regularly, much like the wounded animal, and yet do not die, must have been awesome to primitive peoples. Add to the Bleeding an ability to bring forth other beings with the ability to reproduce themselves, and you have the spiritual basis of Earth-honouring peoples. As the Earth Mother is honoured for bringing forth all the living creatures, the women of ancient traditions were honoured for their abilities to Bleed, reproduce, and tap into the wisdom of the mysteries of life. Our Caney Moon Ceremonies celebrate this connection.

When people live in harmony with the Earth's cycles, the women tend to bleed at the same time. The power of moonlight gently coaxes release from their wombs. Ancient peoples honoured this Moon time by creating special lodges and ceremonies exclusively for women during Bleeding time. In all matrifocal cultures, menstrual Blood has been regarded as a powerful healing essence. Representing a link with the Mother, menstrual Blood was used as offerings to her for fertilizing the fields that grow the crops as well as for bringing forth healing and magical energies. The vast knowledge associated with the healing and oracular powers were gifts received by the women during Moon time, the time when the veils between the worlds are at their thinnest. The future, the unknown, prophetic dreams and visions came at menstrual time and were passed on to the people through the Moon Lodge. In fact, the basis of Shamanism relies on the natural descent into body consciousness that menstruation brings each month.

Along with trivializing our connection to the Earth's cycles, our modern civilization has well-established attitudes and taboos about women's menstrual cycles. Disregard for these cycles, our gifts of knowledge and power, has also brought about a disrespect for women (who create life). On a societal level, women are excluded from leadership decisions, especially those that are of a spiritual nature. On a personal level, women suffer from a new unbalancing disease, PMS, which results from the internalizing of the conflicts and attitudes of a society that tells women that they are inferior because they Bleed and reproduce.

The time for healing both the Earth Mother and ourselves is upon us. Getting in touch with ancient traditions that honour the cycles will enable us to regain the wisdom of the mysteries of Moon times. The visions we will manifest are that women will again be honoured as representatives of the life-giving Earth Matriarch, the healers of the people.

The Clan Mothers of the Caney Circle have been meeting since the fall to re-create the sacred women's space of the traditional Moon Lodges. The ceremonies that we use are a combination of rituals brought back from shamanic work and dreams; the gifts of our Grandmothers. Using the focus of the sacred words spoken at the Moon ceremonies, we honour ourselves for the power and wisdom inherent within during our Bleeding times:

We have within us the rhythm of the Universe, ever constant and steady, the twenty-eight-day cycle of life. We are manifestations of the Cosmic Matriarch, who, together with our twenty-eight-day cycle of life and death, creates the reality we know as existence.

We hold our lodge to communicate with the Grandmothers. They are our ancestors who, through our Blood connections, reach all the way back to Yaya, the first woman according to Taino legend, and her children, the first representatives of the Six Clans of the Taino Indians. The clans represented in our lodge are: Shining Earth, Green Corn, Blue Rain, White Ground Squirrel, and Sky Parrot: with one clan, Yellow Turtle, still unrepresented. We offer the pipe to our Grandmothers, and they bless us with wisdom and healing. Besides personal renewal, the teachings and energy of the Clan Mothers' Lodge reaches out to replenish all of the Caney Circle in various ways. As we expand our ceremonies, we will bring counsel to the Circle, much the same way that the clan mothers of ancient traditional lodges advised their people.

In addition to honouring our Moon times, the Women's Lodge is a space for celebrating other important life cycles of women. These are the blessing of newborn children, menarche rites (onset of menstruation), fertility and pregnancy ceremonies, and blessings for those attaining the status of Elder. These rites of passage were important events for both the Women's Lodge and community focus in traditional Native American tribes. The re-establishment of these ceremonies helps us to value our cycles and the gifts that come with aging. Celebrating again these passage rites allows us to celebrate ourselves.

At the Spring Equinox, the Clan Mothers and all the women of the Circle will again celebrate the secret women's Snake Dance that represents our connection to the fertile cycle of Atabei, the Earth Matriarch. At this time, we will direct our power to the Earth to ask for an abundant Summer. All women are invited and encouraged to attend this sacred traditional ceremony. As the Women's Lodge continues to grow, so, too, will the help of the Clan Mothers to expand the wisdom and power available to the Caney Circle.

✎❧

INTERVIEW WITH MARION Ellis, bioenergetic therapist in her late 30's; Victoria, BC

Bioenergetics simply means body energies. Bioenergetics is a theory of how body energies run through the body in relation to the mind. When our energy gets blocked and caught up in muscular tension, our body and mind have to adapt to the tension. This adaptation could continue for a few months, or for years. Bioenergetics is a way of helping the body release these tensions. What happens is a real healing around the original trauma. It may sound quite simple to heal and recover from these feelings, but, in fact, it takes a fair bit of time to do this work by one's self. It takes continuous effort and persistence to go back and work on that same muscular area and keep working with it to give yourself a chance to let go and free the feelings trapped within.

At this point, healing becomes less of a miracle because you realize you have to experience the pain and emotions over and over again. When the release happens, you also have to overcome the feelings that say you can't express them. That's when therapy comes into play because the therapist is there to help the person relive those moments in a safe way so they don't get blocked again and a complete healing can take place.

Menstrual cramps is a good example of how bioenergetics can be used. I used to have a lot of menstrual cramps. When I started doing the bioenergetics exercises, the tension in the pelvis was released, and, as it was released, the menstrual cramps went away. As I remember, this wasn't enough to get rid of them totally. I also needed an emotional release. With continued work, and more time spent concentrating on the exercise, I started to get in touch with what the cramps were all about. For me it had to do with feeling sexually repressed. As I worked on the release I started to feel angry. Although I couldn't express my anger at my mother, I was an adult still carrying these childhood feelings around in me. This all got very complicated because the anger was directed at so many things. This work took several months and I had several insights about who I was, centred around my sexuality and my source of power as a woman.

For me to be able to express myself fully meant being able to express myself sexually. I still haven't quite mastered it but I feel my sexuality is so much more a whole body experience. The whole trip around my power as a woman and a lesbian has taken me into most of the areas I've had to work on in my life.

PROCESSING CRAMPS, or the Red Blues, Judy Tomandl, dreambody therapist; Victoria, BC

Even as I sit here, I suffer menstrual cramps. My lower abdomen feels in the clutch of something, some figure, some being other than myself. I am literally being grabbed; I bend over and hug myself. In a negative way, part of me is clamouring for care and attention. Well, sure – children resort to obstreperous behaviour if their better behaviour goes unnoticed, or if their attempts to communicate are ignored. If the kids are loud enough, or if my body hurts enough, I pay attention.

A painful body symptom is one way our psyches attempt to communicate with our everyday consciousness. There are ways to work with body symptoms, not merely to be rid of them, but to pay attention and learn something useful about ourselves. Arnold Mindell and others have developed dreambody work, or process psychology, which works to find patterns behind experiences we usually think of as not connected, i.e. body symptoms, dreams, coincidences, relationship difficulties. Process work offers therapists a way to work fluidly in different modes, but it can also be used by an individual to work on herself to gain perceptions and insight into her own unique processes.

Our process oriented way of working with any symptom is to consciously amplify or increase the specific sensation, focusing attention on it, feeling it more. Doing this often results in the body's changing channels of communication, perhaps to a thought or incident, perhaps to movement, perhaps to an inner visual picture or figure.

I am able to access different figures visually and then go into the movements I see them doing. At one time my cramps amplify themselves into a jelly-belly laughing clown; my taking over the sound and movement dissipated the cramps and was fun. Besides, I've been working on developing a lighter approach to life in general.

Another figure I know is a black woman, scantily clad, dancing sensuously. Consciously doing the movements, following my body, helps ease the rigidity, the tightness, and allows me to flow naturally. I am learning to relax and develop flexibility in all areas of my life. Our society inhibits not only a woman's menstrual process but also limits other areas of endeavour. This month when I accessed this dancing figure I was inspired to return to my thinking and research on the benefits of menstruation, a project I've been working on for years.

I've noticed that I always feel full of energy and ready to tackle new undertakings right after my period. I have been working on my own creative process, so I looked up creativity in the thesaurus and was happy to see it connected to nativity, invention, productive, fertile, imaginative, original. To create is synonymous with giving birth, bringing into existence. When my body is not occupied in literally bringing another human being into the world, then my monthly cycle can be a reminder of the creativity available to me which can be used in another channel be it writing, painting, teaching, healing, or being in the world in a new way myself. Twelve times a year I have the potential and opportunity to express myself. Of course, our creativity is available to us at any time, but in our day to day living, when we are coping with the pressures surrounding us, it is easy to lose this perspective.

At my age, with my four children grown, I work to channel this energy, to observe the flow of my experience into revelation and renewal.

INTERVIEW WITH HANA Chucid, psychologist and shaman; Los Angeles, CA

A., my dear friend, had been diagnosed as having breast cancer and was scheduled to have a double mastectomy in less than a week. Her husband F., also my dear friend, attempted humour in the face of his upset. I feel like we ought to cast her breasts in bronze or something! This caught my attention. I didn't know about bronze casting, but I did know how to make plaster casts. I had made many plaster cast face and body (torso) masks for friends, therapy clients, for theatre, and ceremonial and healing work. Why not a "breast mask?" I put the idea to them.

F. was very enthusiastic. "At least it's a positive activity. The creative focus of making a work-of-art provides a way to give positive attention to the whole situation now. It's better than A. sitting around being depressed or trying not to think about her breasts or the operation at all." I agreed with him completely. A., understandably distracted and absorbed in her own feelings and thoughts, went along with the idea carried by F.'s enthusiasm.

On the evening set aside for breast mask-making, the positive focus tone was set when F. provided us each with a glass of champagne and toasted "To life!" A. warmed up to the whole idea as she situated herself comfortably on the couch. All my mask-making supplies were ready and laid out and I began the first step of lightly coating A.'s breasts with petroleum jelly (an important and necessary step, to prevent plaster from pulling on body hairs). At this point F.'s enthusiasm that had spurred the project was overtaken by his own discomfort and upset with the reality of the upcoming mastectomy; he excused himself from the room. A. and I continued.

With the first touch of the plaster coated cloth strips on her skin, A. began to talk. This usually private person began to share stories about breasts – her own, her mother's, her friends. She also began to share feelings about her body, the mastectomy, and thoughts delineating her outlook on medicine, death, life. Mostly I listened. Sometimes I also shared stories, about my breasts, about other women's experiences of mastectomies. Clearly some of these stories and feelings were being recalled, thought about, and shared for the first time ever.

It seemed to me that the thinking, feeling, exploring, storytelling, and sharing that went on was at least as important as the mask-art-product itself. It was the positive focus of the mask-making that allowed us to acknowledge and speak about what was truly on our minds and in our hearts, without sinking into despair.

A. (like everyone else I have every done mask work with) found the whole process very relaxing, including the physical sensation of the plaster against her skin. As the evening went along we were both increasingly enjoying ourselves. From time to time F. would come into the room for a short while. He found a way to be there comfortably and participate by playing artistic consultant, suggesting A.'s next pose or body position for another breast-mask. Towards the evening's end, A. and I were so clearly, visibly enjoying ourselves, talking and laughing, that F. eventually came in and stayed. We made seven or eight masks in all, as I recall. There was her pert, ready for work pose, her what the heck, slouch-on-the-couch breast pose, but her favourite pose, aesthetically speaking, was one in which she cupped her breasts with her hands and her hands are part of the mask.

For a couple weeks, the breast-mask sculptures held prime spots in the living and dining-rooms. Both A. and F. later said it was very important to them to see these masks upon return home from the hospital, post-mastectomy. Later, the masks were brought to a bedroom to prepare for an office staff gathering at A. and E's home. When a staff person wandered into that room and saw the masks, A. and F. called all the women into that room and shared the story of the masks. These women were clearly moved just seeing the masks. They began sharing stories of women's experiences of mastectomy. I was later told that this experience was the first time anyone on the staff had been able to address their own feelings and responses to A.'s surgery.

It is a little over a year since then. The breast-masks now hold prime closet space. F. wants to use one of them as a mold to have an artist cast a three-dimensional resin or plaster sculpture. A. wants this too. As a friend and artist, I was glad to be part of this whole venture. As a counselling psychologist committed to, and experienced in, the use of the arts in sacred ceremony, education, psychotherapy, and healing in general, I recognize much value in the breast mask-making process.

In general mask-making allows "inner" concerns, feelings, to be objectified and therefore more easily "faced." Any major experience of loss evokes grief and anxiety and requires us to re-organize at internal levels (emotionally, psychologically in our world view). Certainly the experience of mastectomy represents one of the more dramatic losses some women must deal with, yet there is virtually no established vehicle or ritual that acknowledges, or addresses, this fact in women's lives. I share the story of breast mask-making with A. before her mastectomy in the hopes that others may find this a useful vehicle through which to acknowledge and address losses and changes-not only in instances of mastectomy, but other significant body-image changes as well. A circle of women I know made a body mask of a full-bodied pregnant woman among them. Subsequently each of the women got to wear, and dance with, the mask. An associated men's circle was given the mask as a gift, a means to explore their own feminine nature through wearing and dancing with this mask.

Mask How-To

Supplies:

Pre-coated gauze rolls (coated in plaster). Available at medical supply shops. This is the same material used for bone-setting casts.

Vaseline and scissors.

Towels and sheets to protect furniture and floor.

Champagne or other positive focus tools, candles, incense, music, etc.

Bowl of warm water. It works best if you dip the gauze strips in warm rather than cool water.

Pre-cut gauze into piles of same-sized pieces. Cut more than you think you need. Smaller pieces allow for more detail in molding the mask to the person's contours. You can also make the mask quite broadly and sculpt the details and exact contours after the mask is off the person.

Directions:

Coat area to be masked with petroleum jelly or heavy lotion to protect body hairs.

Work with one piece of gauze at a time. Dip in warm water.

Smooth out plaster over the strip by running it between fingers. This also squeezes out excess water.

Lay strip on person's skin, smooth and shape it to contours.

3 to 4 layers of gauze is sufficient. In general, make one complete layer before building layers.

The mask lifts easily off the person's body 5 to 10 minutes after gauze has been placed.

If you wish to add more details to it, keep mask damp until just the way you want it to be, then let it dry thoroughly before decorating further. Gluing cloth to the back of a mask adds extra strength, and can be used to tie the mask on the body or face.

If you want to paint your mask:

Acrylics work well. Temperas absorb into the plaster too much. In either case, less paint is absorbed and your mask is strengthened structurally if you first brush it with a coat of diluted white glue (let this dry).

Experiment and enjoy. May the works of your hands and the meditations of your heart be healing.

⚜

COLOURS AND CRYSTALS, G.H., student in her 20's; Pittsburgh, PA

Some time back I attended a lecture about colour and crystals given in our town by Joy Gardener. I found it very interesting. It got me thinking about the subtleties of crystal energy vibrations and colour vibrations on the human body. The only type of problem I've ever had with my periods had been a lot of bloating about a week before I am due. After listening to Joy's lecture I had this flash of insight that the next month I should wear an orange scarf with a carnelian wrapped in it around my belly. At the time, I felt that if I wore orange it would act to dry up the extra water. I was just a beginner at this but it felt right so I tried it.

The next month when I felt the water starting to build up I found an orange cloth and carnelian and tied it around my hips under my clothes. When I put it on, I got such an indescribable rush of feelings. All I know is that the colour and the stone helped to bring up emotions and memories that are very important for my health and growth at this time. As I progress I'm sure I will learn more about energy changes through colour and crystals. I would encourage other women to read and experiment with these energies. I'm not sure what effect they will have on each individual but I do know that my bloating has been lessened since I started wearing my colour and stone. Combined with other forms of holistic healings the use of crystals and colour for health is very helpful.

⁂

AN INTERVIEW WITH SHARON Lesley, psychic healer; Victoria, BC

A lot of people come to a psychic healer because they want to know the future. What that means is that they want to know they are doing okay and things will get better. If I was to say to a woman that she really came for a healing on her uterus, most women would shut down their energy field, whether they realize it or not. The uterus is where we hold our deepest inner pain and it is where we as women feel most vulnerable which is why we experience so much menstrual pain.

I usually begin my session by explaining how I see healing and what I am going to do; this allows her spirit to understand how I run energy through the aura to cleanse and help heal the body.

I also determine how much a woman has invested in being out of her body. If she has a great fantasy about how she sees herself and it is quite different than who she is in her body and how her energy is running, then I have to establish a path energetically for her to realize the difference of being in and out of her body. Women going through a lot of pain, physically or emotionally, don't want to be in their bodies because it is too painful and upsetting, but they can't receive a healing in their body until they are there to totally receive it.

When working with women in such pain, I try to help them get gently grounded and able to run some nice earth energy through their bodies. I do this as I'm talking to them and reading their auric energy. Then I work on the specific issues appropriate to them at the time. Sometimes I will do a hands-on psychic healing if there is a specific physical dysfunction. My healing skills have to do with my ability to channel healing energy into my body. Then, with the patient's help and permission, I focus and direct the healing energy to that part of the patient's physical or auric body needing it. I've found that sometimes people who appear to be most open to psychic healing are the most closed energy-wise, and others who really want a healing don't receive any benefits because they still have something to learn from the situation.

Sometimes illness is connected to a past life event as well. This will show up in a memory form in their aura. This energy isn't needed any longer in their space so I help to clear it away. I work on a physical level as well. I'll go in telepathically and check out the uterus or other parts of the body, seeing which has energy and which is closed. I can then judge the overall strength and health of the body quite effectively. I have to respect each person's healing process. Many times I get information that is really inappropriate to share with the person at the time because they would choose to invalidate themselves with the information rather than empower themselves with it. People need to work towards taking responsibility for their lives and not just blindly accept my truths as their own. I find that once women learn how to channel healing energy, they can heal themselves.

I have never given a healing to a woman that I haven't found major blocks in the uterus or the small of the back. The majority of the women that I have seen have had serious complications with their reproductive system at some time in their lives. This disease in the female centre has to do with the invalidation that we get from society. We learn to dislike our bodies and ourselves.

There are two types of energy – male and female. I believe that the female way to run energy is to take it in, then release it. The male way is to ward off energy and not let it in. Whether we consciously acknowledge it or not, this is the way these energies run through the body. Both men and women can run male or female energy through their bodies and do so at different times in their lives.

The female energy is very sensitive. It takes in and absorbs everything. The path to self-healing for females is being able to absorb and handle all this and then learn to release it again. This process is both literally and symbolically done by menstruation. This menstrual process is having to go through a cycle of change, development, and then being able to release what isn't needed any longer so you can begin again. Women know how to take in and absorb stress but not how to release it after it has been processed. As women we have this creative life force that wants to run through our bodies and revitalize and heal us. If we don't feel empowered enough to release our emotions, that energy gets stuck as stress within us and is used in destructive and self-abusive ways. In order to expand and grow, creative energy needs to be released. It needs to be put out in order to continue the cycle.

The first chakra has to do with physical survival. The second chakra has to do with emotional survival. In our woman's body, these two centres are quite close together. The uterus and the ovaries are connected to the second. Most women, I believe, are struggling to maintain emotional survival and balance in their lives. Most of us are in constant turmoil and upset. This upset comes from not knowing how to separate our own feelings from the opinions and feelings of others.

When we learn to ground ourselves and pull in to our body Earth energy, we reprogram ourselves so we aren't always giving and nurturing those around us until we are drained. We learn to reconnect with Mother Earth and pull in energy and feel nurtured ourselves. We can let go of our negativity and feel nourished. We feel all this in our uterus. When we feel connected to the Earth, we realize She has always been there for us. If we pull up this female energy and use it to balance ourselves and discover our emotional strengths, we can have the power in our bodies to release the disease and our self-abusive attitudes towards menstruation and female genitals.

I personally believe that female energy is as aggressive and asser.tive as male energy, but it gets disguised in unbalanced forms of rage, jealousy, and competition. Behind these emotional states that trap energy in negative ways is energy separate from emotion that can be channelled into healing energy for the body.

In most ancient cultures people realized instinctively that a woman was at the height of her power when she was menstruating. The woman would go to the menstrual hut, not because she was condemned, but because she realized she needed space to discover her power. Today when you hear people complain about a woman being bitchy around her period, it is the epitome of trapped female energy. When female energy doesn't give herself the right to claim her space, then what comes out is the aspect of the bitch. This is very destructive because it locks women into a cycle of anger, guilt, and invalidation. Our body will struggle to get what it wants by negative means if it is denied more positive expression. We must express our need for space through creativity and beauty. If we can't we turn into the Medusa aspect of ourself to get our space. This is also a powerful aspect in the sense that no one wants to hang around with you when you are "vibing the Medusa." The Medusa energy may get you that time to yourself, but once it is there it is probably going to be difficult to soften and love and nurture yourself and not get stuck in the bitchiness. Over time this blocked energy creates disease and illness in the female organs. When you allow yourself to trust yourself, that pain and blocked energy will be released and you can truly be nurtured by the Earth. Only then can you allow nurturing in from any other women. The path to power for women is through connecting with the Earth.

We have been so invalidated by society that it takes time to go away to rediscover these things. I personally believe what Starhawk says. The challenge for men today is to discover brotherhood, learning how to love one another. I think the path for a woman is learning how to love herself, to radiate this love and to be totally selfish, learning to say no.

It is always safe to live vicariously through someone else. Watching soap operas, or surrounding yourself with family and friends who come to you for advice, is the path a lot of women choose. It is safe, but it never gives you space to deal with your own issues and, ultimately, it is self-betrayal. I saw a female client who told me of a very traumatic situation that happened to her as a child. It was a horrific incident that really hurt her as a child yet she told it as an interesting, entertaining situation with a smile on her face. This was the way she had dealt with and integrated this experience. However, as conscious women, we now have to open ourselves up to our feelings and heal. Ultimately, the spirit works through the body, not the mind. We need to realize there is a lot of help available to us from our higher self and the Earth.

I personally believe that metaphysical female energy is evolving at a faster rate at this time than male energy. The way of the female energy is the way the Earth needs to be healed so the more we become empowered as women, the more we help to heal the Earth. I believe this is why the re-emergence of the Goddess is happening in our time.

I work with a lot of women who run more male energy than female. I personally see this as their way of trying to stop being so sensitive. Most women's definition of what is power is their identification with whomever is powerful. Children don't automatically align themselves with who is the most nurturing in their lives but with the most powerful person around them. This is how we survive as children. Usually this alignment is with the father (male energy). The more we ground and run energy, the easier we can allow ourselves to discover our own female energy. This allows stuff to come to us so we can release it. In order to do that we have to give up all our beliefs around wanting to change the energy. This happens the moment we judge it, and when we judge it, we judge ourselves. When we invalidate who we are, our body blocks the energy flowing through us and we create disease.

When a woman has a child she forms a bond of energy with that child which allows her to guess its needs. This is appropriate for a small baby, but many women get trapped in pre-guessing everyone's needs. As children grow they should learn to ask for things for themselves. Women love and nurture often when it is inappropriate, never allowing husband or children to grow up. In the end, no one loves a martyr, and she never gets back the love and nurturing she gives out. This is just another way we avoid looking at ourselves and instead give our power away.

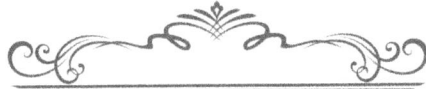

More Blood Rituals

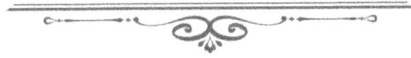

Personal or Group Rituals

A MOON TIME PRAYER
> *Oh Great Mother – Moon Mother*
> *Once more the scarlet river of my Blood does flow*
> *I go to a quiet place to be alone*
> *In the warm velvet darkness I rejoice in my Blood*
> *In the warm velvet darkness I am renewed*
> *I pray*
> *Oh Moon Mother, Womb Mother*
> *As I Bleed*
> *Teach me of your ancient wisdom*
> *As I Bleed*
> *Let me feel the ancient tides within my body, and my womb*
> *Oh Mother give me the strength to look*
> *within and not be afraid*
> *Give me strength to look within*
> *With forgiveness and love*
> *Oh Moon Mother may I know myself*
> *In this Bleeding time and be at peace.*
> *C.W.*

AS I BLEED EACH MONTH I want to recognize and honour, by ritual, the Blood bond I share with all the generations of women throughout time. By doing a ritual to honour my Moon Blood, I reaffirm my link with the past.

I also empower myself to reclaim this lost birthright of Blood, passing it on to my daughter and her daughters in generations yet unborn.

In this chapter, you are given some examples of personal and group Moon Blood rituals. These rituals are merely suggestions, to be used and adapted to meet your own special needs. When doing ritual, I would encourage any woman to always work from her "heart." That means you do what "feels" right for you. Each of us has within our DNA all the information we need to become beautiful, spiritual, and physical beings. We only need to take the time to "listen" to our body cycles. In the quiet of our centre – our wombs – we will hear speaking to us the voice of the universal consciousness that unites all life. By getting in touch with the inner self, that voice of the Goddess, Great Spirit, or whatever you wish to call it, we learn to trust our intuition so that we heal and grow in the way that is right for each of us.

When I create a ritual for myself or others, I draw upon the traditions of both Wicca and my Native American roots. For me, these two traditions blend and enrich each other. These are my cultural roots, and Black and Asian women may wish to add ideas from their own cultural traditions to their rituals as well.

⚬⚬⚬

A PERSONAL MOON RITUAL, Cornwoman

The place and time to do any kind of ritual should be carefully chosen. It should be quiet and free from outside interruptions. It's always nice to get away from it all and do ritual outdoors by the sea or in the forest. That, however, isn't always possible for women with jobs and/ or family responsibilities. Doing ritual in your home can be good, too, because it honours the place in which you live.

I begin any ritual with a symbolic cleansing before entering the sacred space. This cleansing can be done by taking a ritual bath either in the ocean, a lake, or your own tub. (If you do the bath in your tub, I would add salts or sweet smelling herbs for relaxation and scent.) If a bath isn't possible, then a symbolic washing of hands and face is okay. A smudge of sage or sweetgrass or other herbs is equally appropriate. When you bathe or smudge with sweet smoke, what you are symbolically saying to the universe is:

I set aside all my worries and concerns of daily living, I wash them away, I let go of them for this time so that when I enter the sacred circle, my mind and body are clear and open. I am able to be a channel for the spirit power to work through me.

I am definitely not saying that in any way am I dirty, sinful, unclean, or unworthy to meet the sacred prior to my purification. I believe all of us have the Divine within us. I am the Goddess or God, and so are you. There is no need to be ashamed of who we are. To enter the circle, we need only to lay aside our daily routines for a while so that we can tap into the divine energy within us.

After the cleansing ritual, I enter the space I've set aside for the sacred circle. I prepare the space as I wish it to be prior to my bath. If outside, I make a circle marking the four quarters with large stones, coloured stakes, or tiny altars complete with cloths, candles, and other objects suitable to the four elements being honoured. In the centre of the circle I make a larger altar or build a fire. I will enter the circle by the East gate so I leave that marker slightly ajar until I'm ready to enter. When I'm doing ritual inside (in my living or bedroom) the space is much more limited than outside so I usually don't set up four altars around the outside of my circle. I simply add four coloured candles representing the four directions to my centre altar. Wooden boxes or trunks covered with cloth make great altars and your tools can be stored in them when they are not in use. Besides coloured candles, I decorate my altar with statues of the Goddess and God and various items symbolic of the four directions. I often use a tarot deck while in the circle so that also sits on my altar.

For a Blood ritual, I add red candles to my centre. If it seems too cluttered with the directional candles on the altar as well, I remove them, leaving small tokens of their presence instead. For example, a knife in the East, a wand or small plant in the South, a cup of water in the West, and a bowl of Earth or a crystal in the North. In the centre I place my Goddess statue, my Blood sponge, and a sea shell of dried menstrual Blood and/or a cup containing Blood and water.

Now it is time to begin. My first act in any ritual is to ground and centre myself. The most common way to do this is to breathe deeply and imagine roots coming down from your back into your legs and out your feet into the earth. For a man this is the only way to do this exercise, but we are women so let me tell you of another way. Squat or sit crosslegged and breathe into your belly. Feel the warmth growing within your belly, your womb, your centre. Send out a cord of energy flowing from your centre down through your birth canal. Feel your roots coming out of your vagina and going into the earth. Go deep and touch the centre core of living fire that is Mother Earth. Now draw up that warmth and love through the layers of the Earth's shell through your vagina and into your womb. Now allow this energy from your centre and the Earth's centre to flow all through the branches of your body: your hands, your legs and feet, and your neck and head.

Make a shield of protection around yourself as light or thick as you feel you need. Then offer the excess energy outward as you call the four quarters and cast the circle. You are now between the worlds in that place where the individual soul and the oneness of creation can be reunited as they were in the beginning of time.

Remaining conscious of the cord that ties me to the Great Mother, I invoke the Goddess with song. I chant and pray, and as I do, I focus on the Blood of the ancients. That bond of Blood has been passed down to me through the ages of time. I Bleed, yet I am not wounded. I Bleed, yet I do not die. By this magic Blood I claim my woman's power. Because I Bleed, I am woman and Goddess in one. Both creation and destruction are the blessing of my womb. I offer my Blood back to the Earth as a gift of healing. My Blood is my gift. I offer it to the Goddess and paint my face with its rich red colour.

I usually do a tarot reading while in circle during my Moon time. Through the reading, I find where I am, where I've been, and where I may go if current trends continue. I also seek guidance through quiet meditation or crystal gazing. At other times of the month I like to move, sing, and dance to reach this state of awareness, but when I Bleed, I prefer quieter, less strenuous activities. I ask for guidance as to how I can manifest what I've been told during the sacred time. When I Bleed, I feel my link very strongly with all life. At these times I want to make myself clear and open, a channel for receiving guidance, not just for myself, but for my family, community, and the whole planet if need be. My Moon time can be a time for prophecy and vision. It was during menstruation that the priestesses at Delphi made their predictions.

After the work of my ritual has been completed, I partake in an offering of food and drink. Then I release the Goddess (I don't invoke the God during Moon time, though I do at other times of the month) and the four directions, and then I open the circle.

My last act is to return to "normal" space and release my grounded tie with the Earth. For this I usually lie flat on my belly, or touch my forehead to the ground; I relax and imagine all the excess energy that is not needed returning back into the Earth.

To determine if you are doing any ceremony or healing work properly, think about how you feel afterwards. If you feel tired and drained, you were probably not grounded enough so you used too much of your own energy to make things happen. Next time, take more care in centring and grounding. If you feel hyper after the work you have done, you haven't taken enough time to return the excess energy back to the Earth properly. How you should feel is a little more difficult to describe. I personally feel very relaxed, yet I have energy to call upon for any task. I just feel very much alive and in love with all creation.

A GROUP BLOOD RITUAL, Cornwoman

I begin any group ritual by designing the layout of the ritual space so that once the participants enter, their energies become focused directly on the work at hand. That means no idle chit chat occurs once people come into the place where the ritual will be performed. If a ritual is to take place at someone's home, I would prepare the room where the ritual is to occur ahead of time. When participants arrive at the front door, they come in quietly. Then they have two choices. They may go into the kitchen to chat and have tea until they are ready for the ritual, or they may do a simple purification and enter ceremonial space to meditate quietly until the ritual begins. I don't encourage talking until after the ritual has been completed. It has been my experience that many well-intentioned rituals are unsuccessful because energy becomes dissipated ahead of time by participants gossiping while waiting for everyone to arrive. By allowing a quiet time to unwind from the day's events, people are able to devote their energies more fully to the work at hand.

I begin with a grounding exercise. That has partially been accomplished by the quiet time, but something is needed to draw the participants together as a single unit. I would suggest the belly grounding exercise given in the personal Blood ritual. If this doesn't seem appropriate, there are many good books that will offer you other ideas.

In a group Blood ritual, the women are present to honour their Moon Blood and acknowledge the tie of Blood that has united women throughout the ages. This should be acknowledged verbally – always state the intention of any ritual. Then the quarters are called and the Goddess invoked. There are various activities that can be done to accomplish this. The honouring of the Blood can be done by anointing each woman's forehead with a spot of Moon blood. If your circle is reluctant to use actual Blood, then honour your Bloods by sharing a cup of red juice, tea, or wine. Magically speaking, the liquid in the cup can be transformed into the essence of Moon Blood by stating this out loud prior to the sharing of the cup. To symbolize the Blood tie that unites all women, I suggest weaving a red ribbon in and out among the assembled women while chanting a meaningful song of your group's choice. At the end, each woman cuts off a piece of ribbon to tie around her wrist. Time should also be allotted for each woman to share something about her Moon Blood. This could be a first Blood story, a helpful herbal tonic, or a powerful dream that came to her around or during the time of her period. When space and time permit, I always do some type of dance or body movement during ritual. A good exercise is to have women dance out their dreams instead of just talking about them. Dancing out a dream story as it is orally told by the dreamer deepens the experience of the dream for everyone in the room. Lastly, as always, end your rituals by saying goodbye to the four directions and other powers invited to be present for the ritual. Now, when the circle is opened, is the time for food and drink. It is also the time to socialize, if appropriate. Some groups eat while still in sacred space, but I prefer to open the circle first because when eating and talking begins, energies get dispersed and people start wandering off. The next thing you know, some of the women have left without closing that magical door between the worlds.

⚜

M.T., WITCH IN HER 50's; rural California

I lived in the Bay area during the late seventies. I was active with a women's coven there and we used to do Blood rituals occasionally. Nothing very fancy, really. We would just collect our Blood and put it in a small bowl, using it to anoint each other's foreheads as part of a Moon circle. It was very empowering at the time, but now, I'm a bit worried about such things.

In a public circle, you have to be so careful because of AIDS. In a large urban area like San Francisco, everyone is so paranoid about it, and rightly so. I circle mainly with lesbians, which are the lowest risk group, but unfortunately many lesbians take a lot of street drugs so their risk of getting AIDS is heightened considerably. I still really like the idea of anointing and sharing our Blood as women. It certainly made a difference in my life ten years ago. I'm not saying don't use it, but be careful, and choose only close friends with whom to be that intimate – people you are reasonably sure are free from infection.

⚜

MOON, A TRAVELLING woman in her 50's

It was night the first time I really remember celebrating my Bloods. There was a full moon, and I was climbing to the place where we celebrated, which was the breast mound of a hill. I was dressed in white, and as I climbed, I started to Bleed. When I got to the top of the hill, I took off all my clothes and I danced all night. On this particular night, because I was bleeding, I danced in the firelight with my legs open a lot so that I could see the Blood roll down my legs. My dance was a celebration of myself and my Blood. We were all watching the Blood lines. Sometimes the Blood would dry on my legs and crack and start to feel uncomfortable. I would go to my camp and pour a basin of water on my skin to wash off the dry Blood, and then go back fresh for more Blood to roll down my legs. As the night continued, different people left the fire until just my eleven-year-old daughter and I remained.

She was drumming and I was dancing as the sun came up over the night of a Blood celebration.

❧

H.C., PSYCHOLOGIST in her 30's; Los Angeles, CA

At a Long dance ceremonial, on the altar of the Place, we were asked to leave a physical token of our own being. This token served as an offering of thanks to the Spirits of the Place (water, trees, island, birds, ferns, etc.). I was alone in front of the altar so I reached between my legs and smeared my menstrual Blood in a design on the altar as my offering. It felt wonderful to do this. Most people left a piece of hair, some saliva, a fingernail, or something like that. It was the first, and so far the only, time I have ritually offered my menstrual Blood.

❧

C.C., WITCH IN HER 30's; Oregon

There is a nice ritual used by Paula Gunn Allen's group in Oaklands. They give a red flower to each woman on her Moon, and a white flower to each woman past menopause, to honour maturity at each celebration.

❧

S., WITCH IN HER 20'S; Mendocino, CA

Moon Blood is often saved and offered as a gift to the Earth. It is often buried during a solitary or group ritual. I have known women who collect part of their flow for this purpose. Rising time from a night's sleep is the best time to do this because often the Blood flow is heavy for a bit and it may be collected in a jar. Some women have a special flat sea shell they collect the Blood in, which is allowed to dry. The shell is then put on their altar.

❧

M., WITCH; SANTA BARBARA, CA

I know women who can control the amount and number of days they will flow. These women squat over their gardens and let their Blood flow back to Mother Earth. I haven't gotten to that yet.

S.D., FARMER IN HER 40's; Aldergrove, BC

As a farmer, I consider my personal Bloodmeal a very powerful fertilizer. I gather my Blood by using a menstrual sponge, which I squeeze into a glass canning jar that is kept covered by cheesecloth on a high shelf in the bathroom. Each month it dries out and I grind it with mortar and pestle and use it in planting ceremonies. I have also given vials as gifts to other women.

I haven't been doing much solitary ritual lately. Life is too exciting and chaotic. However, I often coincide my Bleeding with our women's Dark Moon circle, and that feels special, to be in a place apart with other women. We've talked about making a woman's retreat place here at the farm – we even put up two trellises as a statement of intention. Getaway? At least it's a start.

K.M., WITCH; OREGON

I sit on the ground with my legs out to either side of me because I need my vulva to be directly against the ground and my spine straight. I have heard that some Indian women do this naked on moss, but I have always had loose clothing on with a pad. Then I close my eyes and say:

Mother Earth, I give all of this most enriching precious Blood to you and I don't want to hold back even one drop.

Then I visualize a rich, thick ribbon of Blood coming out of my uterus and being grabbed by Mother Earth and she pulls on it because she wants my Blood so much. When I picture all this it is like all the kinks in the ribbon dissolve and my cramps go away. (And a lot of Blood flows out too!) I then have a profound Blood tie with my Earth.

A WORD OF WARNING, T.J., witch in her early 20's; rural Nevada

A lot of sisters talk about going out on the land and Bleeding on the Earth. This sounds very idyllic and wonderful, and it is, but let me give you a few words of warning. Be careful about where you go. I tried it, skyclad, in a beautiful sunny meadow, squatting down, Bleeding on the Earth. It was nice, then all of a sudden – ouch! A yellow jacket stung me in the crotch. Oh, my sisters, let me tell you the meaning of true pain! I was transported from bliss to agony in a moment. I could hardly walk for three days and it was very embarrassing to explain to anyone why I was walking so funny. Next time, I'll pick a better spot.

⚜

R.G., HERBALIST IN her 40's; California

I encourage women to use their Moon cycle as a time of ritual, whether they are having their period or not. It is very powerful to create a ritual around the time of one's period every month. One friend of mine had taken birth control pills during high school so her period was gone for years. She didn't mind that at all. As a creative artist, it was just a nuisance and she was glad not to have to deal with it. When she finally realized the importance of her period, she created an elaborate ritual to get it back. This was the first ritual she had ever done, and at the time, the term was still very new. Her ritual involved several other women taking their Blood down to the ocean, marking their foreheads with the Blood, laying it out in the full moon, and sharing the goblet. One full moon later she started her period.

If a woman has a really painful period, she should erect an altar to any one of the Greek or African goddesses with whom she strongly identifies. On the altar, pray every day for power in your fertile being.

A ritual might be the kind of pads you use. If you are sticking stuff up in your vagina to stop the Blood, that can be viewed as a negative ritual. If you are using cotton pads that you made yourself, or bought from other women who have made them, that can be seen as a positive ritual. Sometimes it is simply a matter of establishing positive thought forms. One way to do this is to chart your period. What is more beautiful than to chart your own cycle? This can be elaborate or quite simple. There are some very beautiful calendars available for this purpose.

Moon, a travelling woman in her 50's

I have a red corduroy bag that I keep all my Blood cloths in. When I finish Bleeding, I wash them out by hand to get the Blood out. I give the Blood to house plants or growing plants – wherever I am. I water the Blood down so it is not too strong. Since I've been settled for a while, I have given it to my own plants and they have flourished with this once-a-month fertilizer.

J.Z.N., PSYCHIC READER in her 40's; Victoria, BC

I love the feeling of sitting on a pad and feeling my own flow. I find it extremely sensuous, very sexy and affirming of my womanhood. It just feels wonderful. There is also the sense of cleansing, a shedding of the old, a preparing for the new. There has been, at times, a sense of loss that I do experience as the weeping wound empties itself; not necessarily because I feel the lack of a child. Rather, that I haven't brought something into being during that cycle. I guess I'm just very body involved.

J.B., WITCH; MINNEAPOLIS, MN

When my period comes, I light a large red glass candle that will burn for six days if kept lit. My period lasts four to five days, so it works out well. At night, this little red light on my altar table is comforting and very meaningful to me. When I Bleed I find I like to wear a lot of red and black. I wear my carnelian and copper necklace, or a red belt and scarf with a black skirt or pants. Colour is very important to me, especially when I Bleed. In my busy schedule I don't have time for long involved ritual so lighting my candle and dressing a certain way helps me to celebrate what has become a very important time for me.

T.L., SECRETARY AND witch in her 20's; Colorado

My personal menstrual ritual is to keep a dream diary around that time. I've charted my cycle for years, but only in the last year and a half have I kept a record of my dreams.

I usually Bleed on the full moon starting about two days before until two or three days after. Once I've started Bleeding, my dreams become more vivid and better remembered. At other times of the month I don't remember my dreams for days at a time. I find that I usually have at least one dream around my Bloods that gives me a clearer understanding of something I am working on. Keeping a record helps me to look back and see if a pattern in my life is developing. I have found my menstrual dream diary very helpful. I would recommend it to any woman.

⚬≈≈≈≈≈⚬

S., WEED HERBALIST; Woodstock, NY

I've collected my flow with a menstrual sponge for eleven years, with tampons for fifteen years.

I've been one of the boys; hardly noticed my Bloods.

Lately, I've been close with my Blood-tasting, smelling, feeling it.

Eight months ago I stopped using my sponge.

I let it flow.

I'm still letting it flow.

Sometimes now I need to be alone to let it Bleed.

Often now I need to be away from men when I Bleed.

Now I begin to see more clearly from inside my menstrual cave.

Two nights ago I walked through woods by candle-light

I found a tree curved up from the river's bank,

In a bank of moss, where I sit.

Bleeding.

In the dark.

Silent.

Potential.

I give away potential life.

I give this life to the Earth.

This is the void-birth/death.

This is not life Blood, not new life Blood.

Still, it is life Blood:

Blood full of life:

Potent. Vital.

This is my giveaway, my gift to Earth's vitality, Earth's energy, Earth's potential.

My Moon Blood medicine power.

❧

S.S.W., WITCH IN HER 30's; rural Colorado

A few years ago I started using a Venus sponge to catch my menstrual Bloods. It feels so good inside me. I love my little sponge. I also like the idea of using a re-usable object like sponges or Blood cloths for my period rather than cutting down so many trees to make disposable paper napkins. I collect my Blood on the first day or two of my period when it is at the deepest and richest colour and scent. I don't think it is disgusting at all. After all, our first sight, scent, and taste when we come into this life is our mother's Blood. How could that which represents our love bond with our mothers be disgusting? I gather my Blood in a shell and I offer some to my plants, some to the Goddess, and I dry out the rest to use in magic works of healing. From my menstrual meditations, I created this song which I sing to my sponge when I use it:

Little one from the Sea hold my Blood
hold my Blood,
Little one deep in me hold my Blood
hold my Blood,
We all come from the Sea
And united we can be
Little one I love thee hold my Blood
hold my Blood.
Blessed be

❧

S., HOMESTEADER; RURAL Oregon

Last year at the O.W.L. gathering, we talked about Bleeding rituals, and this is one I wanted to pass on. I went out in a field on my second day of Bleeding with some big sheets of manila paper. I squatted over the papers and dripped Blood on them. Then I folded the papers in half and made blotches. I saved them and use them for artwork to decorate my altar, and for divination. During my monthly cycle, I meditate with them. I find they give me different messages at different times in my cycle. I invite other women to try this and see what messages they get.

A.B., DAYCARE TEACHER in her 30's; Vancouver Island, BC

I get very emotional around the time of my periods. Any little thing can set me off. Lately, I have had relationship troubles. Last month, when my period came, I was very depressed. I was sitting around my house feeling so awful that finally I got up and decided to go for a walk. in a nearby park that has nature trails. I'd never thought about doing a ritual during my period, but after I had been walking for a while I found myself chanting: *She changes everything She touches.*

Later, when I came to a little clearing, it felt very natural to stop, call in the quarters, and do a spontaneous ritual. I sang and prayed and even cried a little. I felt so much better afterwards. Thinking about it later, it seemed so right to do a ritual when I was Bleeding. I'm not sure why I never thought of doing it before. I plan to do something again the next time I Bleed. It feels good to honour that part of my life.

L., POET IN HER 40'S; Houston, TX

For years I longed for a lover interested in tantra or sex magic. When I finally found one, I got more than I bargained for. My sexual experiences with this person, who studied the teachings of Aleister Crowley and practised left hand path magic, were very frightening. I want to warn other women about the possible dangers involved.

Our sexual practices involved marijuana and were based on lust since we were not in love with one another. During our sexual experiences I would reach transcendental heights of passion. However, I would feel completely drained afterwards. It would take me days to regain my vitality. As the relationship continued, I became more and more weak, depressed, and disoriented. Fires started appearing, first in my dreams, then in real life around me. I was constantly frightened. I was determined several times to break off with him, but was drawn back every time.

I went to my friend Cornwoman for help. Her prayers and the herbs she gave me helped a lot. We consulted a Native Shaman who discovered that my former lover had actually marked my body in three places to hold my will subject to his. I had to go through a lot to be rid of the influence of this person on my life and personality.

My advice to other women is to only have sex with people whom you love, and who love you, and do not use drugs. If you are having good sex, you will feel full of energy and vitality afterwards. If you do not feel that way, examine what is happening to you carefully, and don't be afraid to ask for help.

❦

B.C., WITCH IN HER 30's; Pittsburgh, PA

I make love to myself for my own pleasure and also as part of my ritual practices. I use this sexual energy in different ways. I can redirect my thoughts during orgasm towards healing or towards some creative project I am working on at the time. I can also use my bodily fluids (my cum or Blood) to anoint my ritual tools or to anoint a charm or amulet that I could give to another woman to help her own healing process. Used in this way, my body's liquids are strong medicine. Especially so at the time of my periods, when I can easily mix the red and white flow.

❦

F.D., STUDENT IN HER 20's; Seattle, WA

A friend in Seattle told me that her women's group got together and rented a little cabin up in the mountains to use as a retreat by their members when they are menstruating.

I am impressed with their energy and determination. It wouldn't cost much if several women got together. Women I've talked to think it's a great idea, but around here, if you don't get a government grant to do something, it doesn't get done. You just talk and wait.

❦

R., STUDENT IN HER 20's; Tacoma, WA

At a political meeting I went to recently, a woman from one of the African countries spoke about the tremendous economic strides women were making in her country. It was interesting to me that one of the major reasons she gave for this change was the opening of a sanitary napkin factory in her area. She claimed that now women didn't have to spend one week of each month in a tent sitting over a hole in the earth. Now they could be just like men – get a good steady job and work all the time, without taking off time for their periods as they used to.

Later, when going home, I remarked to another witchy friend how odd it was to hear that woman speak. So many women I knew yearned for a tradition like that of the Moon Lodge where they could go and get away from it all at that time of the month.

It's sad in a way that in Third World countries where women still have a traditional culture of sorts, instead of supporting their culture, they want to throw it all away for a box of Kotex.

⚜

R.T., WITCH IN HER 40's; Vancouver Island, BC

Our women's group has thought up a new kind of idea for a very mobile and high tech menstrual hut or Moon Lodge. Let me start at the beginning …

A while back, one of our members read an article called The Menstrual Maze. The article explained how some women in New Zealand had created a maze representative of the female reproductive organs by using fabric and other natural materials. Women walked through the vagina, into the womb, and so on. The article claimed the experience was very meaningful for the women who had experienced it. They even held a ritual inside the womb.

It seemed like a wonderful idea. Our women's circle talked about it and decided to try to create something like it. We all started checking around fabric stores and second hand stores for cheap red materials. It took us several months to gather enough, and once we had it we weren't sure what it was we wanted to make. Then we got a great idea. Eva's brother's six-man dome tent had been ripped up pretty badly by a bear on the Pacific Rim. We decided that we could use the tent as a pattern and make another tent out of the red cloth for our Moon Lodge. The tent was a dome so it looked like a uterus. It was very portable and we could all sit inside if we wanted to have a ceremony. It seemed like a great idea. We could pack up the Moon Lodge and take it with us to summer gatherings, or individuals from our group could borrow it for their own private retreat when they were Bleeding.

It has worked out well, but not quite as we first thought. First of all, the tent the bear wrecked was grey and maroon. We found our cheap material wouldn't work for a new tent so we patched up the one we had and bought some red waterproof material to make a weatherproof fly to cover the tent so it looks red and is also weatherproof in bad weather. The cheaper, red material already gathered was sewn together and staked out around the Lodge like a small maze. This provided privacy from passersby. When women entered, they went through a couple of turns in the maze before coming upon the open clearing and the Moon Lodge. We had a fairly large area enclosed outside the Lodge so we could hold rituals if we wanted. We furnished the Lodge with a couple of foam pallets with red, plush covers, several big pillows, and a small altar table with a diary should someone wish to write down her feelings while resting in the Lodge. We have considered cutting out a hole in the centre of the tent floor so we could dig a pit in which to Bleed. Right now we just dig a pit outside.

We used the Moon Lodge at one gathering last summer. It was a great success. For most of the four days, women just came and went as they wished, staying a while, then going back to the big camp. We hung a Bloody napkin at the entrance of the maze so that no man would mistakenly wander in. On the last night of the gathering, we held a Blood ritual outside in the clearing in front of the Lodge. We passed around a cup of wine to symbolize the Blood of the Goddess and consecrated our foreheads with menstrual Blood. In the firelight we danced to the drums until almost dawn. This was our longest and best Blood ritual. We hope to do others next summer.

<hr>

MASKS OF POWER, CORNWOMAN

As I placed the mask of the Dark Moon Woman over my face, I felt her power flow through me. That is the way of masks if they are made properly with love, concentration, and many prayers. A spirit will come live within the mask so that the user will feel the spirit's power while wearing it. When any spirit comes and honours your sacred things by leaving a little of itself with you, this power carries with it certain responsibilities. In the olden days this was so and all the people knew that. Nowadays, many people who seek power, seek it for power's sake. Selfishly, they do not understand that such gifts are to be used for the good of the people, not out of fear or for personal gain.

I understand these things about my masks. Before my masks were made (I have two at this writing) I had dreams in which these spirits came to me. The masks were made over a long period of time. That way, their creation had time to be nurtured and grow to maturity. My masks are made out of plaster strips soaked and placed to dry over my own face. Then the masks are painted, varnished, and a headdress of hair is added. It is a simple technique that anyone can do, yet if done with craftsmanship and love, they can be as rich and powerful as any wooden mask. No matter what the material, it is the spirit of the mask and how it is used that is important.

My masks are kept in their own baskets. They are not hung in my living-room for anyone to stare at. They are only brought out on special occasions when their power can be witnessed and do good in the community. I also offer them food and drink occasionally in honour of the spirits who live within them. To have created the masks does not mean that they belong to me alone. They belong to the people. I am only their caretaker. I have a responsibility to dance in them, or use them in other ways to help heal the people and keep them strong. They are not mine to be used disrespectfully, flippantly, or selfishly. This is the way I was taught by the Elders of my people. I pass it on because many haven't had the chance to know these things as I have.

To dance in a mask or speak through one at a sacred ceremony is a very special thing. It is difficult to explain in mere words. It is like allowing the self to drift away, and yet it is not, because the power flows through you like a current. It can be healing for you, the dancer, and for those who witness your dance. I believe strongly that the ancient arts of mask-making and dancing with masks should be revived and used more often in the pagan rituals and Blood ceremonies of today.

H.C., PSYCHOLOGIST in her 30's; Los Angeles, CA

In the Jewish tradition, a woman marks her Blood flow through a shift in life-style. The basic premise of the shift is an abstinence from sex. Some women even go so far as to refrain from any physical contact whatsoever with their lover during this time. As far as I am aware, there is no traditional ritual practised during the actual Blood flow period.

Upon completion of a woman's Blood flow time, she traditionally does a mikveh, which is a ritual bathing. Most orthodox synagogues will have a mikveh bathhouse available for Jewish women wishing to keep this practice, but I have been observing the practice of mikveh for years and rarely go to a built bathhouse. Rather, I follow the basic guideline that a mikveh body of water must be fresh and large enough to support fish life. That means the ocean and most lakes and rivers are perfect natural mikvehs. Sometimes, in the middle of a Canadian winter when I lived in Calgary, my bathtub became my mikveh, though a mountain river is a tremendous context for a true-rebirth cleansing mikveh!

Usually, mikvehs are witnessed by one or more women, though occasionally my lover (a man) and I have witnessed mikvehs for each other. At other times the trees and river are my witnesses. To perform the mikveh a woman first prepares herself physically, mentally, emotionally, and spiritually. Preparation is two-thirds of any powerful transformational practice. Preparation can include bathing for purposes of physical cleansing, clipping nails, meditating, praying, dancing, putting on special ceremonial garments, or setting aside special garments to put on after the mikveh is completed. Usually, a woman immerses herself fully in the waters a minimum of three times; some like to do it three times in each direction. This total immersion recreates the waters-of-life of the womb, and the whole ritual re-enacts a birth.

I like to think of the idea that, although we were born through the physical womb in pain, each time we do the mikveh we can heal the pain of physical incarnation through choosing a mikveh intention-focus to be born in joy and with ease. Sometimes I choose a focus for my mikveh, deciding beforehand Who-Within is dying to allow Who-Within to be born; between immersions, I name the One-within-Who is Being-Born during the mikveh itself. After at least the first immersion, a traditional blessing is said, such as:

> *Blessed are You, One Who Was-Is-And*
> *Always Shall Be, Ruler of all Universes*
> *who makes us holy with Your*
> *gifts of Life and who requires*
> *of us to serve Life in holiness.*

In Judaism, the one name for The Divine which takes the feminine form is Shechinah (the ch in the middle is the back-of-the-throat sound in Hebrew). Shechinah is understood as The Divine manifest in all forms, all physical beings-including our bodies. So, we are Shechinah, we immerse in Shechinah, and we serve Shechinah in serving Life. This is a little known little talked about aspect of Jewish tradition. Certainly it is appropriate to call upon, honour, and celebrate Shechinah as part of any sacred Blood ritual.

I believe that the misunderstandings of both the abstinence from sex during menstruation, and the ritual bathing afterward, comes from a misunderstanding of what is meant by the term unclean. This term is found in Biblical discussions of Blood and Blood rituals. This misunderstanding has to do with the broader disassociation in today's world of Death from Life, and the consequent denial of Death and practices which acknowledge Death as a natural part of cycles. As I understand it, what comes down to us translated from early Hebrew as unclean means specifically ritually unclean or impure. In turn, unclean here means very specifically that which is associated with Death, that which is not fully Life, Life affirming, and Life creating. To acknowledge and respect both the Death and Life parts of the Story, Jewish tradition embodies many practices that require the ritual separation of that which is Life from that which is Death. Although menstruation reminds us of our life-giving potential, actually and symbolically, each Blood flow can be seen as a mini-death in that it is the loss of a potential life. Even if a woman has no intention of becoming physically pregnant, the Blood flow time is commonly recognized as the end of the cycle, not the beginning. Since, in this sense menstruation is a mini-death, many practices follow from here. The life-style shift of no sexual relations is consistent with mourning practices; at a time of letting go of life, you do not engage in creating new life (actually or symbolically). The mikveh, at the end of the Blood flow, symbolic mourning time, then marks the beginning of a new cycle, a new life, a re-birth.

❧

THE ART OF EARTH SPINNING, Cornwoman

I call myself an Earth spin dancer. What do I mean by that? It is difficult to describe this type of dancing without seeing it, but I'll try. When I dance I spin Earth-wise (counter-clockwise). I imagine myself as linked to the Earth, Herself. I have this image in my mind of a woman spinning and spinning, surrounded just by fire. In short the Earth, Herself. As I spin, I send my energies down, down, boring into the Earth. I tap into Her enormous power reservoirs at the centre and draw the energy up into my body. I spin faster and faster. When I feel the time is right, I move my hand and twist my head as I spin to release that energy into the space where I wish it to be.

I have a Sufi friend who also Earth spins. Though her techniques are not quite like mine, the feeling she taps is the same – a joyous reunion with the Earth.

Many people feel that if they spin, they will get dizzy and fall. Not so. I have never fallen, and no matter how fast I am going, I can always stop on a dime. I am always in control of what I'm doing, though an onlooker may not believe that anyone could spin so fast and be in control. I try to spin in a small area, though I don't hold one foot on the floor at all times as do Sufi twirlers. The other thing I never do is try to focus on an object in the room as do ballet dancers. When you Earth spin the purpose is to sever your ties with everyday reality and go off into a trance. If you need to focus on anything while you are learning this technique, focus on your hand, allowing everything else around you to become a blur of motion.

I began this type of spinning as a child. I am legally blind, so could not do a lot of the sports that other children did. Though I never thought about it at the time, I guess it was a way of combining daydreams with exercise. My mother was afraid of my spinning. She thought it would single me out as different and weird. Though I never stopped completely, for many years I spun only occasionally and in secret.

When I discovered the Craft, my spinning took on another deeper meaning. I began to realize what a wonderful gift it was. I am a firm believer in using the total being when doing ritual or spell work. This is the wisdom the ancients knew. Combining body, mind, and emotional energies creates a much stronger energy field than just using the mind alone, as in meditation. When I spin I use all of myself. I can go deep into trance and go to deeper levels of awareness. Or I can tap into Earth power and direct it to some good purpose or just use it to heighten energy in a room where a ritual will take place. I am sure there are other uses for my spinning that I will learn as I cast off my mother's warnings and predictions of doom and allow my gift to be used.

⁂

EARTH SPINNING-A BLOOD Ritual, Cornwoman

Last summer, at the full moon in July, I was Bleeding. My cycle skips around a bit now that I am approaching menopause, but at this time it was right on the full moon. Prior to this time I had been feeling quite down. My four boys were out of school, bored, and driving me crazy. I also felt stuck, spiritually and emotionally, with no end of the tunnel in sight. I wanted very badly to do a ritual, but I was having trouble finding a quiet space and the time to do it.

The night of the full moon I went to bed about ten, feeling totally drained and exhausted. Around three o'clock in the morning, my eyes popped wide open. I rolled around in bed a while, but couldn't fall back to sleep. Finally, I got up and went into the living-room. I drew the drapes, lit some candles, and put on some low music. After a time I began to chant softly and play my drum. I felt this was the time I had been waiting for to do a healing, energy moving ritual. I got up and arranged my four candles in the four directions: yellow-East, red-South, blue-West, and green-North. In the centre I placed a white candle and a statue of the Goddess. I stripped off my gown, panties, and pad. I wanted to do this ritual skyclad. I began by smudging myself with sweet grass and sage. Then I stepped into the circle and chanted, called in the directions, and invoked the Goddess. I sang and chanted for a while longer, but I couldn't raise much energy because my chanting and singing might wake my family. So I stopped. What to do? I put on my mask of the Bleeding Goddess, began to breathe deeply, to feel the air go deep into my body, into my womb. My womb felt tight and hard, it throbbed slightly, allowing my flow to come more freely down my legs as I swayed gently back and forth. I enjoyed feeling it and watched its patterns. I took off my mask and placed it near my altar. I took some of my Blood on my finger and painted the face of my Goddess statue. I told her that this was my gift to Her, the sacred Blood of my body. I told Her how grateful I was for my life and how with the gift of my Blood I offered my life in service to Her anew.

I painted my own face and breasts. I felt very strong. I began to spin, my hands moving, acting out my words as I spun. I can't remember all I said or did after that, but I can give an idea, a flavour, of what was said and done. It went something like this:

I am the Earth spinner haya!
I am the weaver haya!
I create it and I cast it
I create it and it is real
I spin it and it is real
I go down deep into the womb of the Earth
and draw up the Energies of change
I go down deep into my own womb
and draw out the Energies of change
Haya! do I feel it Haya! do I touch it
Haya! do I know it
From this full moon's Bleeding to the next
I create a change in my life
I use this energy for my healing
From this full moon's Bleeding to the next
I use this energy for the good of all
Grant to me oh Mother Earth what I need
not necessarily what I want
Grant that I may know what I can give
to the greater good in return
I spin it and I weave it

I heal and I touch it
I create and I cast it
By the power of the Goddess
And by the power of my womb
So must it be.

As I stopped spinning, I redirected the power through my hands, then grounded it. I felt very energized and content. By this time it was growing light in the East. I bade goodbye to the Goddess and the four elements. I then put my tools away and took a bath. I felt very relaxed, and afterwards, fell back to sleep immediately.

Since that time, things have been changing, slowly at first, but faster now as we go into fall and winter (my special time of power and creativity). I had used my spinning in group rituals before this, but never in my private rituals. For me it is the best way I know to pull up power and use it for healing and good. I hope this story will encourage other women to try spin dancing themselves as a way to become more in touch with the Earth Mother and their own bodies.

<hr>

THE MOON CIRCLE WOMEN; Victoria, BC

The Moon Circle Women had been together for three years when emotional problems and group commitment became real issues for us. We started out high with everyone focusing on the rituals. There wasn't any processing of our personal lives at all. When these issues started coming up, it was felt that the group wasn't an emotional support group, and if support was needed by the members, then the goals of the group needed redefining. It was a hard time for us. I think the hottest issue at this time was whether we should be an open or closed group. This caused a lot of conflict. We wanted to keep the group fairly small, but we each had one or two friends we wanted to invite to our meetings. One night we put all the members' names in a basket and picked one name and that person's friend could join. It was fascinating to see that no one felt good about this, not even the woman whose name was picked. We then decided that we wanted to be a closed group. At that point we felt more safety in our group than is possible in an open circle. We decided to have open circles occasionally, when we could invite our friends, but most of our meetings would be closed.

It takes time to move together and grow as a group both emotionally and spiritually. When a new person is added, the safety level drops until the new person is absorbed. For me, the Moon Circle was a real challenge because I've never been that intimate with anyone before. It's the only place where I can work on real gut level honesty. The other thing I see about our group is that it is a place to take on different roles and challenges with the support of others. Things are easier for us now and we can really concentrate on deepening our experience with ritual. At the full moon in January I realized that this was my third year of commitment to the group and it felt good.

Our rituals are usually at the full moon, or sometimes at the new moon, but usually once a month. We all lead pretty busy lives so our communications have to be clear in order to get the date and times straight. There are nine in our group, and usually six or seven show for any given ritual. Lately we've been talking about meeting twice a month; at the full moon for ritual and at the new moon to hang out and talk about our lives, drink tea, and massage each other. This way when we meet at the full moon we could move right into our ritual instead of spending time talking. You have to be clear to move into ritual. We've had some pretty frustrated moons when we've started the ritual and someone starts processing what's happening in her life. The ritual gets sidetracked by helping that person with her problem. Because we act co-operatively, with no one acting as high priestess or facilitator, all of us have to take responsibility for getting the ritual back on the track. One of the exercises we've been trying lately is to have one or two of us take over and plan and facilitate the ritual for that moon. It seems to be working out well. With different women taking on the role of high priestess and directing the flow it keeps things moving.

We actually had a non-verbal moon once. It helped us focus on not talking and to get us out of just sitting around and chatting. It was a good exercise.

Another good exercise we tried we called the Ovarian Palace. It was adapted from an Oriental system of energy that we changed around to focus on the ovaries as the place of creative power. We began by drawing the energy into our centre by contracting the vaginal muscles. We drew up the energy and then transformed it into a stone. We crystallized the energy into a jewel. Then we empowered the jewel by taking it on a journey. We put it in the Earth, in water, and then in fire and air. After the journey, we walked back into the Ovarian Palace where we were met by guides. The guides asked us what in our lives was preventing us from owning this power, this creative energy? What prevented us from taking this energy out of the palace to use in our lives? We did this at the solstice, a full moon, and we called it drawing down the moon. These are the darkest days of the year, when the Earth draws down the energy into Herself. By opening ourselves to Her, we can be freer to explore our unconscious. We are able to bring it into the light of understanding. This Ovarian Palace exercise was symbolic of the time of year, as we moved back towards the light.

There was also the feeling that we wanted to tap into our creative energy and to use the group to help us do more and get out of our rut. We wanted to make the point that our creativity lies in our bodies and we need to bring it up more fully in order to use it.

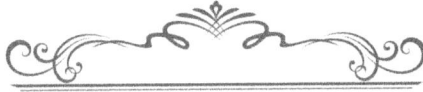

Creating the Red Flower

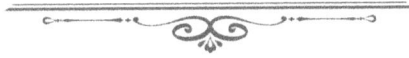

Poetry and the Literary Arts

IN MY MOTHER'S GARDEN there is a red flower growing
its essence is bright and fragrant
it is strong and alive
Each month the moon waxes
and the flower bursts forth in radiance
singing the praises of creation
Each month the moon wanes
and the flower folds in her petals
to look within, but still singing her ancient song
K.P.

CREATIVITY IS LIKE the waters of an ancient underground spring. When drunk, its water is infinitely satisfying and refreshing; but too often, its course runs too deep to tap easily.

Over the years, as I've become aware of my spiritual path, I've learned to pay attention to my monthly cycles. I have found that within my body is the gateway to this hidden well. As I learn to use my Moon time as a time of contemplation and spiritual growth, I find it easier to taste the waters of the creative springs. All things are connected. By paying attention to, and going with, the flow of your personal tides, you will open many new doors helping your creativity to flower.

Whatever your interest – art, music, politics, or housework – using your monthly energies will enable you to blossom in unimaginable ways. I hope these pages will inspire further growth in this sadly neglected area of our lives.

⁂

THE SHAMANIC DRAMA,
Tzuniguah Women's Circle; rural BC

Our women's group has been experimenting with prolonged in-depth rituals for large seasonal gatherings. We prefer participating in ceremonies that last several hours, or even a day or two, like the ancient ceremonies. During the course of the rite, our group likes to enact Shamanic dramas that help channel and portray the divine forces present at these sacred events.

In ancient Greece, actors saw themselves as instruments to be used by the divine will during a performance. In our work we hope to recreate and pass on this ancient honoured tradition.

I would like to stress from the first that what we do is not psychodrama or any other type of group therapy.

When we are preparing for a performance, many unresolved emotional issues come up and are worked on, but in the performance itself, there is no room for personal crap if the actress wishes to manifest the sacred. Our aim is to become a clean and open channel for the Goddess or God to enter and use as they will.

As we work together, the plot outline is developed, and characters take on form and substance. Through our dreams we are directed to make certain masks or costumes that will reflect the power of our rite. All this takes time, concentration, and effort. I've been assured by Native Elders that this is the way to go about such things. After working this way for a while, I feel the difference. It makes it incredibly hard for me to go to most pagan events that are planned the night before or the day of the actual ritual. They are so shallow in comparison to our work.

The style of our performances seldom varies. There are one or two narrators who weave the telling of the story – somewhat like a guided visualization. In a sense, we expect our audiences, or witnesses, to participate with us in enacting the tale. Masked dancers act out the deeper feelings of the tale with mime, dance, and occasional speech.

Accompanying both dancers and storyteller is the chorus, which begins the play with the beating of a drum, a sound that will continue like a heartbeat throughout the performance. The chorus sings, chants, and plays other musical instruments at appropriate times during the play.

From this description, it may sound like our women's group consists of about twenty or thirty women; not so. At any one time, there are only eight to ten of us. The storyteller remains the same, but dancers, chorus, and technicians are interchangeable. The plot outline for any performance is quite structured although the storyteller's words may vary. Our costumes are elaborate, but our props simple – we can perform anywhere from a large living-room to an ocean beach.

Our performances rely on group energy and a light trance state which channels the divine. As you can imagine, this is all quite intense. So far, we've only done five performances like this in two-and-a-half years. I wish we could do more, but modern life is too busy and stressful. Alas for the good old days of temples and kept priestesses.

One of our most successful dramas is called I Dream of Red Roses Bleeding. The story outline and chants were spirit gifts given to one of our members in dreams and meditations. The tale is of a young girl's growth into womanhood where she meets the Goddess as she begins to Bleed for the first time. I can't share the actual script here because it's too long, but here are a few samples of the chanted songs from the play. I hope this explanation will encourage more women to develop their own ceremonial dramas in future.

⚜

CREATION CHANT
by Tzuniquah
From her womb I was formed
in fertile darkness safe and warm
Tasting Moon Blood deep and red
down the passage was I led
Falling, falling, falling
down the river's flow
Falling, falling, falling

through the gate I go

DARK WOMAN CHANT
by Tzuniquah
chorus
Dark Moon Woman
Bloody Woman
You are, Red Woman
a very special part of me
verse
For years I did deny you
So many fear your ancient power
But now I am one with you
I'm reclaiming my past
repeat chorus
verse two
Like the Tides of the ocean
my body is one with the moon
both creation and destruction
are the blessings of my womb

COMMUNION CHANT
by Tzuniquah
Hear me, oh my children
Drink of my red wine
Wisdom, healing
Blessings of the Blood
I am the gateway
So spoke the Goddess
Reclaim your birthright
Bless your heart, your soul
Your body with Moon Blood

⦅❈⦆

ROSES CHANT
by Tzuniquah

In the night, in the night
in the warm velvet night
I did dream, I did dream
and in my dream she did sing to me
Come away, come away
Come to where red roses are Bleeding
Peace will you find there
Healing will you find there
Come away to where red roses are Bleeding

⦅❈⦆

RED TO REMIND US
Colleen Redwoman, witch; rural W. Virginia

Dracula drinks it
the patriarch curses it
Some women can't stand the sight of it
Some men commit mass human sacrifice
in Blood-letting wars
The power makes us faint
So we teach our daughters
to hold it in
to throw it out
to take the cure to relieve them of their burden
I wear mine
like woman's warpaint
I fight the myth
I give mine
in birth
in death
I am anointed through the passage
Deep red magma

I am erupting passion
for life's sake
for sacred life
I am earth rivers rising
emptying into heart
into red clay womb
I give mine back
I give mine in Moon time
in the name of the Mother
The grail's first wine

RED BLOOD MOON – A Woman's Ritual
Colleen Redwoman, witch; rural W. Virginia

Vivid Red
Vital Force Red is for Passion
for action
for faith Red is the colour of Heart
I Bleed in the East
where the yellow flicker comes
where the earth is warm
where my love is open
like a red rose petal
our waters mingle
I spill my Blood for love
I Bleed in the South
where the red hawk comes
I warm the rain-soaked ground
like a brooding hen
I incubate the earth
the embryo potential
I am alone
I am naked
I Bleed in the South for life

I Bleed in the West
where the black crow comes
red berry juices
sweet ripe offering
red stained body
against the green summer grasses
I give my Blood to war no more
I shed my Blood in peace
I Bleed in the North
where the white dove comes
where the earth is cold
I surrender rites
I mark the earth
and she remembers
I pour my Blood like holy wine
I nourish the earth
who has nourished me
I Bleed in the North
in Thanksgiving

MENSES
Dalla
The Blood Tide ebbs and
flows within
moonful to the heart's thunderpump

MEDICINE
K. L. Patriarche; Victoria, BC
She is in the hospital
She is going to have her ovaries removed
She must do this because they will hinder the drugs they
will use against the cancer in her bones, her body.

She has had her breasts removed, one at a time. She may
have tumors in her lungs.
They are taking out her ovaries because they will work
against the treatment
They must take her apart
She will work against the treatment
her body is her enemy, She is her own doom.

THE CYCLE
K. L. Patriarche; Victoria, BC
the Blood the death the clean one the
swollen sphere the Blood the death the
new one the Blood the Blood the white Blood
the Blood the Blood the death the Blood the
death the freedom the dead.

MY TIME IS COMING
K. L. Patriarche; Victoria, BC
My time is coming,
Creeping in black alleys,
Hiding.
Sun is retreating now
Climbing into the earth to rest.
I am extruding long amoeba fingers
Into the night. I am slithering
Through daytime into
Cool covering night light.
Moon is growing full in sun-
Lacklessness.
In moon's borrowed light I firm into shape of woman; like
Others, covered with skin, like
Others, dark eruptions in me

Spill on fertile ground.

✦

K.L. PATRIARCHE; VICTORIA, BC

the Blood on the thigh is the Blood of the child
the birth of the man the Blood is the birth
the Blood on the thigh is the Blood of the child
the Blood of the dead the Blood is the birth
the Blood on the thigh
the Blood on the thigh
the child is covered with Blood
the new Blood
the Blood on the thigh
oh and the women cry out at the new one
you have Blood on your thigh
the life has come out of you
the Blood on the thigh
the Blood on the thigh
the child is covered with Blood
the new Blood
the Blood on the thigh
oh and the men cry out at the new one
you have Blood on your thigh
the new one has come
see the bare face of the new man above
the Blood on the thigh.

✦

TWENTY MONTHS LATER
K.L. Patriarche; Victoria, BC

I am covered in mucus, sweat, Blood.
I am swimming in thick juices.
My womb is swollen and empty,
My belly gross and silvered.

I am covered in snail trails, red snakes.
I am heavy breasted
My milk spills from my nipples.
My tears spill from my eyes.
I am covered in thin milk, thick tears.

CELEBRATION FOR MENSTRUATION
M.A., witch; California

I invoke the Triple Goddess.
By the power of three times three,
Maiden, Mother and Grandmother,
bless me.
Dark Moon perception Bleeding
into unconscious Sea
Nine Virgins!
Ecstasy!
Her skirt is the net of light
that captures and holds her truths.
My intent is perfect identity.
In the accumulated night
conscious gives quiet birth
The breeding salmon of wisdom run
Nine powers!
Change!
Darkness gathers in her womb.
The sun spins red around her.
The milk of her wisdom is red, is Blood,
is white as starlight.
In her dark all things
are as big and important
as children.
My skill is perfect clarity.
The sleeping intellect sloughs ignorance

through the living womb
Nine priestesses!
Awareness!
She walks in the sea.
She sees the stars by day.
She owns the night.
My end is infinite peace.
Purity, enlightenment and dissolution bless me.

ART OF THE SACRED,
Interview with Ann Rosemary Conway

It has been ten years since I discovered the Goddess, or should I say, She discovered me. Being an artist, I was drawn at first to Athena because there were such wonderful sculptures made of Her in ancient times. I could see in these statues that She generated a lot of honour and respect in the people that worshipped Her. She is the Goddess of Creativity, and for any artist it's always a struggle to get an idea into an outward form, such as poetry, drawing, or sculpture. Athena is the Goddess who brings things to fruition and so I was drawn to Her; and She, in turn, lead me into investigating many other goddesses – mainly Greek and African.

Looking back, I can see that things began to change for me when I read Merlin Stone's book, *When God Was A Woman*. At that point, I dedicated myself to the Holy Mother, and from that point on, She took care of me. I decided to go on a journey throughout the Middle East, to look for the lost goddesses, and reclaim them on every level of my life. I realized what a loss we women have suffered by not having access to these feminine deities in our lives.

At this point, as I prepared for my trip, I became drawn to Artemis. For me, She is the adventurer, and I was adventuring into whole new areas after being a victim of circumstance all my life. She appealed to me because She represents the power to choose. She takes aim, sets Her bow, and goes after what She wants. I decided to focus on taking a trip to see as much of this ancient art as I could, in person. I wanted to go right away, but my children begged me to stay until they finished high school. They used to chide me about doing things backwards. it's the children who are supposed to leave the nest, not the mother. When I did go, the trip was incredible. I took thousands of slides and made hundreds of sketches. I travelled all over the Mediterranean and the Middle East for several months, and the power of that experience is still with me in my life.

Right now, the Ashanti Goddess, Ohemma, is my favourite. I saw a statue of Her in an art gallery on my birthday. I saw this marvellous moon-shaped Goddess. I was drawn to the whole essence of Her. She was sitting on a stool holding Her swollen belly, and that symbolized, to me, new life and creativity. All these symbols run together for me. When I dream of babies, I get a lot of new creative ideas, so I bought Her and She has taught me many things since coming to stay in my home. I've begun to study primitive art. I'd read some books before, but when Ohemma appeared, I knew why She was there-to help my creativity in this area blossom. One of the ways it blossomed being some very successful prints of this Goddess herself.

It took me quite a while to find out the name of this old Ashanti Goddess because so much knowledge has been lost. With Her, and the other Goddesses, I've done a lot of research to find out their ancient names and how their stories have been changed by patriarchal cultures.

To give you a good example; recently, in our local newspaper, there was an article about ancient stone carvings found here on the West Coast of BC Well, damned if the article didn't describe a West Coast Indian carving as a man holding his penis. I just couldn't let that go by, so I xeroxed the picture of the carving, and pointed out the large vulva and the child's arms and legs. I sent it off to the paper and the museum saying that, unless phalluses now grow arms and legs, I doubt very much that their interpretations are accurate. I've been studying this for ten years and had my conclusions verified by a noted archaeologist in Vienna, but I've received no comment from the paper or the museum about my letter.

I think it's very exciting that we have our own Goddess here on the coast, and sad because we are being denied Her by these male scientists who don't want to recognize women's importance in primitive societies. My next pet research project is to try and discover Her name. Names are important because when you name something, you invoke its power into your life.

All over the world you can find evidence of how these ancient carvings and paintings have been misunderstood by men. It's very frustrating. I think it's very important to have images of the Goddess in Her many manifestations around us; visual stimulation really stirs the pot of our creativity. I never get tired of looking at them because I know they are feeding me at an unconscious level.

As an artist, I think it's important to gather all this information, nurture it a while within, then bring it forth changed into a new form that everyone can enjoy. Art is a very external symbol of very internal processes. About 1,000 years ago, as patriarchal cultures grew in strength, art lost its original function and became merely decorative.

Art's true function is to invoke certain powers in our lives. It's forgotten that the images you surround yourself with invoke certain things in your life. These kids that walk around with knives dripping blood on their T-shirts are, in fact, invoking violence into their lives. It's sad. Why not invoke good things in our lives by surrounding ourselves with positive images of the sacred?

We do create our worlds – I know that from my own life. I find much of modern art very shallow. These artists have missed the point of art's function. Their work is dead compared to pieces thousands of years old in museums that still radiate power. I hope more women will become interested in creating this sacred art. As of yet, the climate here isn't right – there aren't many angry-women artists yet, and that stage usually precedes the sacred art.

Part of the problem is making art for money. This doesn't interest me because I've always seen my art as a tool of my own personal growth, not something to please the market. A while back I created five large circular paintings, four feet in diameter. Four were for the four elements and four seasons, with the fifth being the centre.

This project took me over a year to complete. I worked on each one during its season, drawing on the energies of that element and season to create the shield as I worked. Some were easier than others to make, but it was a time of tremendous personal growth for me as each one came into being. I felt like a totally new and transformed person after that. Now I use the paintings as part of my altar when I do a ritual. They are very powerful.

Art should be a part of our lives and spiritual growth, and as more women discover the Goddess in their lives, I am sure we will see more of this powerful inspiring art to guide us.

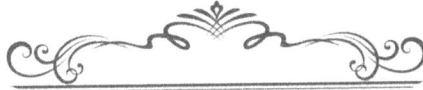

When Blood No Longer Flows

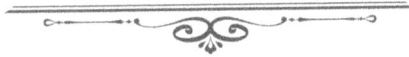

Menopause – Hysterectomy

THE OLD ONES
the old ones
the winnowing ones
the spinner
the one who grinds
the distaff, sinister,
the weaver
the weaving woman
the ones who watch me
the gathering woman
the sewer
the one who grows
woman in the skies
the ones who stoop
and whisper
the strength is in the Blood.
K.P.

MENOPAUSE IS WHEN THE Blood no longer flows each month. In this way, women throughout the ages have ended their childbearing years. Over time, the menstrual periods become less frequent, and finally stop completely. When this happens, a woman flows naturally into a new state of being, her cronehood.

Today there is another more abrupt way of ending the monthly cycle. A hysterectomy is an artificial menopause; it abruptly stops menstruation which, at the time, may seem to be a blessing, but emotionally, and later physically, its effect on a woman's body and psyche may be drastic.

Unfortunately, doctors are encouraging more and more women to submit their bodies to hysterectomies, many of which are totally unnecessary.

By whatever means, natural or artificial, a woman comes to that state when the Blood and the power of the Blood are held within her, she needs to pause and ask herself how she can best use the gift of the Blood. How can I love myself, my family and community, and the living Earth?

In these pages, women who no longer Bleed tell their stories. I can only listen to these stories and say, Grandmother, we honour you and need your wisdom in our lives. It is my hope that in this sharing, older women, and all women, will come together to share with and support each other in love.

⚜

I.C.J., CRONE AND GRANDMOTHER; Vancouver Island, BC

When I was younger, I had the power to create and nurture life both in my womb and without. I believe our gift and responsibility as women is to teach our families how to love and relate both to each other and to the world around them. If a woman is in tune with her body, she can intuitively know a whole lot. Women are the creators and civilizers in this world. Women know instinctively how to nurture life and live in harmony with the Earth and its creatures.

On the other hand, I believe men are natural fighters and destroyers. It is our job as women to domesticate and civilize them. When I was younger, my responsibilities in this respect were to my family. Now that I am older, my responsibilities as a teacher are to my community and the planet as a whole. At no other time in our history has the need been so strong for women to speak out for the Earth and for peace.

This speaking out is the job of the grandmothers, the white-haired women. We must create more of this feminine consciousness in the world, or our grandchildren may not have a world to be born into. I believe this is imperative.

As post-menopausal women, we no longer shed our Blood, but hold our power and our Blood within us. We can, if we choose, be incredibly strong women. We must do this for the good of all. We must stand up and say no to pollution and the cutting down of forests. We must say no to war and bloodshed. When a woman learns to use her Moon times for creativity, prophecy, and vision, she has strength later in life to use her gifts for the good of all.

When I look around me and see all the poor old people, both men and women, wasting their last years in sickness and self pity, I feel so sad, and a bit angry, too, that society doesn't recognize what a valuable resource is being lost.

I feel like I just began to really live when I turned fifty. As older women, we need to get together as well. We need to support and honour ourselves, and by working together, help create a new world of peace and love for our children and grandchildren.

⟨⟩⟨⟩⟨⟩

CRONE CIRCLE WOMEN, women in their 50's and 60's; Victoria, BC

1.

I guess, like the onset of menstruation, I was looking forward to growing up again, going on to a new stage. I'd missed a few periods, but they always came back. One weekend last October, when my period was due, I had no Blood but instead had hot flash after hot flash. It was quite a tense weekend for me. Since that time I haven't had a hot flash or period.

2.

I believe there is a certain power in hot flashes. There is a purpose for them. In the old days I'm sure women knew that purpose, but we have lost that ancient wisdom. When you fight hot flashes and tense up against them, they, like menstruation, can be more uncomfortable than necessary. In my house, one advantage to hot flashes is warmth. It is very cold in the morning, so I wait in bed until I feel a hot flash coming on, then I get up and get moving. It's great, and it saves on the fuel bill.

3.

Women go through menopause differently from each other. Some have an easy time of it; others find it very difficult. My mother had a very hard time. She was institutionalized for a time and I guess I've always had this little fear that I would go crazy too. So far, however, except for a few flashes, it hasn't been so bad. Vitamin E is supposed to help some women, but it hasn't helped me. Maybe I need a larger dose.

4.

My mother is the model for my cronehood. It was wonderful being with her and her friends, all of whom were in their eighties and all very active. Until she died, my mother always planted a big garden, with rows of wonderful vegetables. Everyone who knew her was amazed by her vigour. We all wished we had half as much energy, as well as her positive outlook on life. Before her death, she told us what she wanted us to do for her funeral celebration. We weren't to be unhappy. We were to have wine to celebrate her passing and that's what we did. In making a centrepiece for the funeral table, I took all kinds of little trees and plants and vegetables from her farm. Later, I took some of these things and transplanted them in my own yard. Over the years, many of the trees and plants have died, but I still have one tree that we took with us when we moved. I want to start seedlings from that tree in order to pass this tradition to my children and grandchildren. To my mind, this is symbolic of a family putting down its roots.

5.

I have a different picture of my mother now because she has grown and changed so much in the last few years. She has let go of a lot of things and so have I. We're working through many things in our relationship that we never could before. I see her now as such a dynamic person even though she has been assessed for extended care. She doesn't actually look so great, but if I close my eyes, I feel a much larger energy field around her.

6.

Before my mother died, when she still knew who we were, I began to wonder if a part of my mom had already gone off somewhere to work on another plane. I could see it in her eyes, sometimes, that although she was still hanging on to life and to us, she had already partially left us. I think she wanted to go, but maybe felt we wouldn't let her go. A big part of growing old is letting go of your children, husband, friends, and what you thought was yourself.

7.

I was living alone after my children were grown and I decided I would explore the healing properties of water to induce orgasm because of the physical arrangement of my shower. I have a hose that goes down the wall that made it easier to experience this. The first time it happened I was facing North when I found that this was a really gentle and soothing way to have an orgasm. The first time it took a long time to reach orgasm because my body didn't quite know what to expect. At first I noticed the soles of my feet began to burn as the energy shot up to my head. It was a very grounding and empowering experience. I felt this incredible spiritual connection to the universe. I then turned to face East, South, and then the West. I discovered I could have several orgasms at one time. Returning to the North again the circle felt complete. Sometimes it feels like the bathroom is filled with angles, and frequently I have had the most profound visualizations doing this. It is such a connection with the cosmic universe. I know that there are a lot of women living alone for one reason or another, and I think this is a wonderful way to feel connected with the universe and to feel like you are a part of the whole thing. I make my bathroom into an altar. I light candles, play music, and anything else I can think of to feel in touch. I started doing this ritual about eight years ago before I was introduced to any type of pagan knowledge. It just seemed like a natural thing to do, stand and face the four directions as I had an orgasm. I felt it was an offering.

8. Up to this point in my life, it seems to me I have always been, and still am, a mother. Although my children have left the nest, I am still the mother they come home to with their troubles and joys. I also have my older parents to care for and, in a sense, I've become their mother, too.

Since I'm in the middle ground, I've begun to assert myself a little more in my relationships. I need to go into myself more. I have to take time for me before I can give outward again. Consequently, I'm not always available like I was before.

If a woman doesn't have a steady job, she can find herself being a mother forever. If she's still in the home and available, she'll be the one called on, the one automatically jumping to serve, if she isn't careful.

9. I feel in the middle. I am older, but still middle-aged. My children are grown and on their own. They don't need me, but I can see that my mother does, and I need her because I've had very little contact with very old women. I think I need some lessons on how to grow old, or maybe, how not to grow old. It's wonderful for me to be with my mother. I've only now been able to view her as a person in the last seven or eight years. Before that, she was my mother. To get to know her and to forgive her has been a very affirming experience for me. I find that, because I don't have to prove myself to her constantly, I am a person, too. She is so open and generous with me. I've never experienced that before, so it is really wonderful. I know I'll cherish these years always.

10.

When I went through puberty, I sweated a lot, so it seems normal to me that it should happen again at the end of the menstrual cycle. The menarche is gaining hormones while menopause is their loss. If that loss is sudden, it is more traumatic. If gradual, then the transition is easier. I've noticed that thinner women seem to have more severe symptoms because hormones are stored in body fat. When one doesn't have that extra to draw upon, as your body adjusts to a new state, it is more extreme.

11.

I experienced more psychological traumas with my periods than I did during menopause. My thirties were especially tense years. I had a lot of PMS, not to mention the upsets of a divorce and being a single parent. My children were young and there were lots of problems.

12.

After my husband died, I stopped having periods very abruptly. I guess the shock just stopped everything. I had no real problems with it at all.

13.

I haven't had a period for about a year now, but each month I still seem to go through PMS even though I'm not Bleeding. My body is still hooked into the same cycle. It's more a psychological tension than a physical experience. It may be connected with the moon's rhythms. I have to start keeping track. I know it's my pattern, but I haven't checked out where the moon is when it happens.

14.

Since I began menopause, I have had a lot of problems with insomnia. There are several little rituals I do to help me sleep. I fix herb teas to relax me, do lots of relaxation visualizations, or read. I wonder about the spiritual reasons for this. For me, it's a wonderful freedom: I live alone now, so I can do what I want. It's a very empowering time. I should check to see if my insomnia is connected with the moon. It's an interesting idea. Perhaps as we lose our own bodily cycle, we take on the larger cosmic cycle of Grandmother Moon.

J.L., LIBERATED WOMAN; Vancouver, BC

When I think about getting old, I think of the word freedom. When I was a girl, I was controlled by my family. As a young woman, I experienced some freedom when I went away to university, but I didn't know what to do with it and gave it up too quickly for a husband and children. For years, family responsibilities kept me tied down, and I had little time for myself. Those were good years, but I'm not sorry they are gone. Now I'll have time for myself.

Recently, my twenty-five-year marriage broke up. After the kids were gone, my husband and I had little in common. We are still friends, but we go our own ways now. I'm a little lonely, but I'm learning to handle it.

It's a wonderful feeling, freedom. It's great being old; not at all what I expected. I feel such a sense of detachment, and yet compassion, for my children when they come to me with their problems. I can listen, yet be objective. I've been there and know that whatever it is, it will change with time. After all, nothing lasts forever.

V.N.S., GRANDMOTHER in her 60's; Atlanta, GA

When I was in my teens I worried about growing older and passing through menopause. I listened to my mother and her friends talk about the horrors of hot flashes, menopausal depression, and other complaints. In my mid-twenties, I moved away from that smothering small town atmosphere. I read more and began to think for myself. I went through a period of rebellion and my family was quite shocked and scandalized by the new me. I smoked, swore, and wore clothes my family didn't approve of, but over the years I've come to terms with that. It was a necessary part of breaking away from my roots, but really just a stage. As far as my body is concerned, one of the advantages of my rebellion has been that I never accepted all those tales about menstruation and menopause. My periods never hurt, so why should menopause be a problem? It's a natural occurrence for a woman, just like menstruation and childbirth, isn't it?

I'm sixty-five now and still going strong. I stopped Bleeding about twelve years ago with almost no problems. I account for this in several ways. Physically, I eat well and am pretty healthy and strong. I'm a little stout by today's standards, but that's not a bad thing for a woman of my age. I've read that heavier women are less likely to get osteoporosis and some of the other ailments of old age than thinner women.

Physical health is important, but attitude is just as important. Over the years, I've watched my mother, sisters, and other relations. I know what kind of lives they live, and I know the kind of health problems they have. I can't prove it scientifically, but I believe it nonetheless – one's attitude about being a woman affects how the female organs function. If a woman sees herself as a breeder and nurturer, like my mother and older sister, then going through menopause can just about drive you crazy because they don't have interests apart from their family responsibilities. I've always worked – had to – and I still work part-time. I enjoyed my children well enough, but I never let them become my whole life. I'm glad that part of my life is over. It's nice to come and go as I please and do pretty much whatever I want. If I could give some advice to the young girls coming along behind me, I'd tell them to be proud of who they are. Enjoy being a woman. Take each stage as you come to it and enjoy it fully while it lasts, but when it's time, let go and move on to the next stage in your life. Life is always full of surprises, sweet and sour, good and bad. They are all a part of it. Enjoy it all.

P.L.S., RETIRED LEGAL secretary; Baltimore, MD

It makes me angry when I see women like Tina Turner on TV. She's almost as old as I am, and yet, she walks around in mini skirts with her hair dyed like she was twenty-five. I'm not against mini skirts or dyed hair as such, but if you are fifty+, what's wrong with looking and acting your age? There's something sad about a woman trying to be forever young. Men grow old and so do women, so why can't we women grow old with dignity?

Our society places too much value on a youthful appearance. It's a shame all those poor old souls are wasting away in nursing homes because no one cares. Older men are thought of as distinguished, but an old woman is just a hag. I'm proud to be old. I did a whole lot of living to get here and I'm not ashamed of how I look, and, if there are some who don't like me the way I am, that is their problem.

I always taught my children to respect old people because some day they will be old and then they might want a little respect, too. When a society doesn't respect its old people and seek their advice on things, that is a society well on its way to ruin and destruction.

⁊⁊⁊

P.P., COMPUTER PROGRAMMER in her late 40's; Vancouver, BC

Sometimes it is stressful for me to have my old parents living with us. My father has diabetes and is very hard to live with. My mother constantly tries to feel needed by doing things for me and my daughter that we don't want or need. She has ruined so many of our clothes that I have to lock up my dirty laundry so she won't do it for me. I always feel in the middle, a mother to everybody-my daughter, my grandchild, my parents. Even though it is difficult, I keep my parents at home because I want my daughter to have a role model on how to behave. Our cultural and family traditions are important and I want her to see that. Your parents make sacrifices to take care of you when you are young and, in turn, you have to make some sacrifices to take care of them when they are older. I think it is terrible to put old people away in nursing homes.

It's not all bad. My mother and I have grown closer than ever before. She had a hard time understanding why I didn't marry my daughter's father because in our culture a single woman is nothing. I didn't because I saw what my mother put up with. Now that we are older, we can understand and appreciate each other's choices in life.

⁂

J.N., MUSIC TEACHER in her late 40's; Victoria, BC

I'm forty-four and I think I'm going toward menopause. I feel awful asking my doctor about menopause because I feel like I don't know anybody going through natural menopause. All the women I know have had hysterectomies, and they've gone through a kind of artificial menopause, or have been on hormones, so I don't have anybody to talk to.

Because I have no role model to follow, I feel as though I am on an island and going through this thing alone. I certainly wouldn't choose to be in a situation like my friends who have had hysterectomies and are using hormones. On the surface, it might sound like a good idea, but I don't think so. It's difficult to get the hormones to balance and a lot of women suffer accordingly. My friends look well, but when they tell me what is really going on, like the problem with cramps, it's not a desirable situation.

They may have had no choice, because of tumours and other problems; however, many operations are done without sound reasons. Statistics show that doctors' wives and nurses have the most hysterectomies. I think this is because they are tied into the medical system and they believe what the doctors tell them. There may be other options, including natural ways like vitamins and herbs. If you have a tumour and you're not sure if it is cancer, there isn't much choice. I certainly would look at every other option before I went ahead with the operation.

⁂

INTERVIEW WITH HERBALIST, Rosemary Gladstar; California

It's embarrassing and interesting to me to be asked to teach workshops on menopause. I think it is good to share information, but it's not so good to share information that one has not experienced. The information I present on menopause comes from having watched women go through it and knowing what herbs worked for these women. I have read the literature, but I haven't experienced it, and I always feel a little bit of a fool. Someday I hope these classes are taught by menopausal women because they know what they are talking about.

The primary system I work on during menopause is the endocrine system. Through this, I work on all the glands of the body with a group of herbs that are also associated with the liver and the immune system – specifically, however, these herbs feed the endocrine system. The herbs I use are the seaweeds because they are so high in trace minerals. I also use ginseng, an excellent herb for menopausal women, and I use Eluthero, and Russian and Chinese ginseng. Eluthercaucus is really excellent, but the Chinese ginseng – the panaxting – is also good, as is dongquai, chasteberry, and sage. One of the best remedies I know for hot flashes is motherwort and sage in a tea.

Huckleberry leaf is another herb that is really good for the endocrine system. A lot of herbs are used for this method of focusing on the adrenal glands because the adrenals are made to take over the hormonal function of the ovaries once the ovaries have stopped working at menopause.

Basically, menopausal symptoms and adrenal stress are almost identical. I assume that the reason women from highly civilized cultures suffer from menopausal symptoms is because, by the time they reach their early forties and fifties, the adrenals are so stressed out they don't have the ability to respond when menopause sets in. They don't have the ability to take over the ovarian function. If the adrenals, as well as the whole endocrine system, are kept nourished, the menopausal woman will have an easier time of it. If we begin to focus on the endocrine system in our thirties, then when it is time to enter into our old age, our wisdom, we can do it more graciously and without stress.

A good adrenal formula includes sage, raspberry, peppermint to taste, and lots of motherwort. I would give chasteberry, dongquai, and/or ginseng for adrenal stress. Also include borage with the sage and motherwort mix. This is good for courage and the heart. Licorice root, wild yam, and one of the cohashes are often used. Always use liver herbs, too – like burdock and dandelion root. If one mixes a cleanser and a builder into a formula, make sure they are harmonious. A good mixture would include yellow dock, burdock, dandelion, and dongquai.

HONOURING OUR GRANDPARENTS,
   Spider, Caney Indian Spiritual Circle; Pitsburgh, PA
   On the mantle in my room sits a small altar with pictures of my grandmothers. It is to this place l bring flowers on special occasions and pause for a few moments each day to ask for guidance. It is in this way that I keep alive the spirits of my grandmothers by honouring our connections.
   In the Caney tradition, the spirits of the dead are called "hupias." In many ways, the hupia is the spirit of that person we once knew. After death, as the person's body returns to the Earth, the hupia also slowly fades – or the hupia can be kept alive by our constant practice of remembering and honouring these persons.
   My flower offerings and small gifts, as well as smudging the pictures with sage, opens up an avenue of communication with my wise grandmothers. They, in turn, talk to me through my dreams and shamanic journeys, giving me spiritual gifts and practical advice. Or, as I am following my daily routine, I will feel the presence of one of my grandmothers and, suddenly, the answer to a problem becomes clear.
   By honouring our grandparents in this way, we honour our Blood roots all the way back to Ia Ia and Guaguiona, the ancient humans who parented the six clans from which all human life descended. In this way, we honour the wisdom of the past, allowing it to remain in our lives. There's no need to feel cut off from our ancestors. They're still with us, waiting for us to recognize their presence. In whatever special ways we choose, grandparents are happy when we open to the presence of their hupias, and will bless us with their wisdom.

N.W., ON BECOMING A Woman of Power; Tucson, AZ
   When I was younger, I fasted many times and prayed for a Spirit Dream or some other guide to aid me. Alone in the vastness of earth and sky, alone by the water, I felt open and unprotected. I could feel the land, the sky. All who choose this path of knowledge and who feel these things are both awed and afraid. That is why spirit helpers come to aid and protect us.

When I fasted, spirit guides came to me. I learned many things which helped me to understand myself and my relationships with other human beings around me. Yet always the fear, the little fear deep inside, held me back. There was always a door I dared not open, depths I dared not swim, because in those depths and behind those doors lay forces so strong that all my being would be needed to face and survive them. To become a Woman of Power, I would have to let go of everything. I would have to take the ultimate challenge and stand in that place where there are only three choices possible: death, madness, and that blending with, and control of, the Elemental forces which make one a true Woman of Power. Many years of living are needed to have enough personal power to stand in that place. Rare is the youth who can make the journey and survive. Once, I held Hecate's weed in my hand. Among the old people, this plant was used as a plant of power, but the user must have the power to blend with the plant's spirit or the weed will kill them. I held the plant in my hand with reverence. Her spirit questioned me; I drew back. I was not willing to die; I could not surrender completely. At the time, I had young children still at home and, although I hungered for that gift of power, I wasn't willing to die. Who would take care of my children? So I pulled back. It wasn't time for me.

Now my children are older. They are on their own and so am I. Someday, perhaps in the spring when the frogs sing their awakening songs and the Earth is renewed, I will go alone to that place between the worlds where the three choices lie. And then, we shall see.

⚜

CRONE RITUALS, CORNWOMAN

On examining cultures around the world, we notice that although First Blood rituals abound, little is done to honour a woman's passage through menopause into old age.

Throughout history, poor nutrition and health conditions meant that few women lived through menopause to reach old age so there was little point (culturally speaking) in creating a ritual to honour the event. Biologically, the task is not much easier. While going through menopause, many women skip a few periods then start menstruating again. It is often difficult for the woman herself to know when her cycle has completely ended. For these reasons, and others, there seem to be no rituals that mark the end of the menstrual cycle. Today a woman can expect twenty to thirty years of life past menopause. That is an unbelievably long time to enjoy life free from childbearing responsibilities. As women rediscover their ancient spiritual roots and begin to heal themselves, the need to create for ourselves new rites of passage will be felt; rites honouring the crone, the wise old grandmother, whose wisdom will help guide us all into a new age. To aid in this process of new beginnings these few rituals are offered. They are but the beginning. it is up to the wise old ones themselves to carry on from here. Just as we younger women are reforming into Moon Lodges and women's circles to heal and explore our women's spirituality, so too, the grandmothers are coming together in healing and wisdom, to support each other and offer guidance to younger women and to the community as a whole.

At this time in our history, we need the wisdom and guidance of our old wise grandmothers.

E.W., GRANDMOTHER IN her 60's; Northern Minnesota

When I had one whole year without any periods I knew my Bleeding cycle was finally over. I have been involved with Wicca for several years and I wanted to do something to celebrate this passage into a new stage of my life. There wasn't a lot of tradition even in Wicca for me to draw upon so I wasn't sure what to do. At first I was very frustrated by this. I wanted some form already there that I could tap into and use for my own purpose. My woman's circle offered suggestions, but nothing was quite what I wanted

Finally, I realized that one of the tasks of this passage was to create my own ritual. When we are younger our families, husbands, or society tell us what to do. With this passage through the gateway of menopause, I now realize it was up to me to choose my own path and my own celebration. It was like feeling I'd finally grown up. So I sat down and planned the whole thing out. I allowed free rein to my imagination.

Five days after the full moon in July, I began my croning ritual. Several friends and my son and daughter joined me at our summer cottage by the lake. We had a lovely time. We sang and danced a bit and my women's circle fixed a delicious meal. As it grew dark, we had a candle-light procession down to the beach where I took leave of them. Then my son, a friend and I got into a canoe and began rowing away from the shore. The others called their goodbyes as we drifted away into the night. I was in a long green dress with flowers in my hair and around my neck. I had a thick wool blanket around my shoulders because the night was chilly in the woods even though it was summer. I was going to a small island out in the lake where earlier that day my son and his friends had set up a tent and made camp for me. As part of my self-styled passage into cronehood, I chose to go on a three day fast and retreat in this isolated place. As we rowed away, I could hear my friends singing on the shore. Then, holding their candles high, they returned to the house to continue the party. In a few minutes we landed on my little island. It isn't much bigger than my backyard at home, but I felt very safe about being there. There were a few trees for shade and a nice flat rock to sit on and look out over the lake.

When they were sure I was settled okay, my son and friend left me and rowed back to the cottage. They would come for me again at sunset of the third day. I sat up for most of that night watching the moon on the water. It was a wonderful feeling. At dawn and dusk and moonrise each day I was there on my rock. I prayed to the Earth Mother and the Goddess to bless and guide me along my new path. I chose to do this retreat at the time of the waning moon because it's the time of the crone. I wanted to feel that moon energy within. I wanted to experience how I would relate to the natural world now that I was no longer a Bleeding woman but one who holds on to her Blood, keeping its power within.

I slept most of the days preferring to save my energies for the nights when Hecate rose high in the dark sky. It was the most wonderful and magical time in my whole life.

At sunset of the third day they came for me. My friend and daughter brought new clothes for me to wear. I bathed in the lake and put on my new robe – black with silver trim around the hood and sleeves. As a surprise they gave me a little silver headband with a crescent moon in front. We rowed back to the shore where my friends and family were waiting to welcome me back as a crone. With candles aglow, we went back to the cottage and gave thanks to Hecate for her many gifts. I told of my dreams and insights while on the island. Later we feasted and danced until dawn.

RITES OF PASSAGE: CELEBRATING the Crone, Maggie

All over the world, in every time and place, people have celebrated Rites of Passage – the landmarks of life. We celebrate the birth of a new baby, and welcome that child into the community. We celebrate puberty, graduation, marriage, even retirement, but as far as this writer could discover, no society has ever celebrated menopause, unless the women alone observed it and left no record.

One of the nicest things about the Old Religion is that older women are valued and respected. No longer either sexy or fertile, we are despised by the material western world. At an age when a man achieves distinction in his career, a woman sometimes feels her life is over.

We decided to put an end to this foolishness. Our Women's Circle celebrated a croning by ritually sharing the forty-ninth birthday (seven x seven) of one of the sisters. We focused our ritual around the symbol of the gate, marking the passage from the realm of Selena, the full moon, to that of Hecate, the waning moon, Lady of Wisdom and Magic. There was a willow tree, sacred to Hecate, in the garden, so the gate was installed beside it.

In order of age, the sisters arranged themselves in a circle. We talked about what we were doing and why, chanted, and made music. Then the oldest woman present quietly slipped through the gate and closed it behind her. The sister whose birthday it was took leave of each in turn, widdershins around the circle. She was escorted to the gate where she buried an infertile egg and a vial of menstrual Blood on the threshold before passing through. She was greeted on the Hecate side by Eldest Sister, who covered her with a black shawl and took her out of sight.

After the ritual there was a feast. One of the skills that improve with age is cooking so it was a very fine feast indeed. Next year there will be two Elder Sisters waiting to greet the next one who will pass through the gate.

Loving thanks to all the sisters who helped make the first recorded croning.

Grow old along with me,
The best is yet to be,
The last of life, for which the first was made.
Robert Browning

❦

CRONE CIRCLE WOMEN, women in their 50's and 60's; Victoria, B. C.

On my fiftieth birthday, I decided to have a croning ritual for myself. I invited everybody to come in white, wearing flowers in their hair. This was one of the nicest rites of my life. Here were all my friends in white, flowers in their hair, and holding candles. The men wore flowers in their beards. It was lovely. I was amazed that everyone took me seriously and did as I asked.

I had no sense that I actually passed through menopause. I just wanted to do something to celebrate my fiftieth year, something with honour and dignity rather than the usual indignity of growing old.

❦

CRONE EMMA JOY'S FAVOURITES; Hornby Island, BC

Luna Cease – it is time for public recognition, and, therefore, let each woman celebrate luna cease on her fiftieth birthday, whether or not Blood still flows from her womb. Each woman must know that, as on the day of her Menarche she was blessed, and as on the day of her first orgasm she was twice blessed, on this day she is thrice blessed.

On her fiftieth birthday, let the woman clothe herself in blue and let all who love her surround her. Let her be seated on a great pillowed divan in their midst. Let the one she holds close to her tell of her accomplishments, and let all the children call her mother, for all women are mothers of the Earth and shall be honoured, equally.

Let a young daughter place on this woman's head a garland of flowers saying:

Our great Mother is the source of all life, unto Her both the flow and the ebb, both the waxing and the waning are holy – therefore on this day we honour you ...

Another "croning" was given by our Seaside Lesbian community. We honoured three women who turned fifty this year with a ceremony at Hallomas. A crowd of thirty-five formed a circle in crone-ological order, with eight women over fifty. As these women enter the third phase of life – Maiden, Mother, Crone or wise woman – we celebrate their aging.

We saluted the four comers and "smudged" the room with sage and cedar, a Native American custom for clearing negative energy. We passed a cup of juice around the circle, making our thanks and wishes aloud or silently. Miraculously the cup did not need to be replenished; our version of "loaves and fishes", someone chuckled. We sang our favourite songs and chants and did a banishing ceremony.

Each woman wrote something she wished to rid herself of on leaves cut from construction paper. We wadded them up and cast them to the floor. Two of the new crones swept them up with their new brooms, while the third tended their burning in a tiny cauldron. We presented the new crones with garlands of leaves and flowers, crone jewels (crystal pendants), and special robes. Our youngest member, the nymph for this occasion, read a powerful poem while all tone-chanted. We asked for healings, protection, guidance, and expansion for the coming year (Hallomas being witches' New Year). Afterwards, in the kitchen, we had popcorn and hot cider, and many hugs for our three new crones.

⁕

GRANDMOTHER LODGE, Brook Medicine Eagle; Helena, Montana

I come speaking to you as Buffalo Woman of the North, your Elder Sister. I am Earth Woman, deep rooted in the land, and I am Spirit Woman, carrier of the Great Mystery. Today I come speaking of the Grandmother Lodge, to the women within it, and to all those who would know about their function. Women, awaken and see, for you approach this lodge. Men, awaken and listen, for these are your Elders, the keepers of the Highest Law.

This Grandmother Lodge is the lodge of the white-haired (wisdom) women, those who have gone beyond the time of giving away the power of their Blood and now hold it for energy to uphold the Law. When we choose to wrap ourselves in the robe of an Earthly body, we also accept a charge, a responsibility, a gift which is to be shared. As we choose a woman-body, the charge we accept is the nurturing and renewing of all things. And the tool we are given is Creator's one law, You shall be in good relationship with all things and all beings in the great hoop of life. (The Law of Good Relationship.) Creator's gift to us as women is an inborn knowing with regard to all the aspects of relationship. This is awakened, developed, and deepened through contact with those in our society who model this aspect. Then our duty is to share these deep understandings with our brothers and our families, that harmony and peacefulness might reign among us.

And when our Elders step across the threshold of the Grandmother Lodge, they become the Keepers of the Law. No longer is their attention consumed with the creation and rearing of their own family. In this sense, they have no children, and in our ways those who are not parent to any specific child are parent to **all children**. Thus their attention turns to the children of All Our Relations: their own children, the children of their friends, their clan or tribe, and the children of all the hoops: the Two-Leggeds, the Four-Leggeds, the Wingeds, the Finned, the Green-Growing Ones, and all others. Our relationship with this great circle of Life rests ultimately in their hands. They must give away this responsibility by modeling, teaching, and sharing the living of the law in everyday life to men, women, and children that all might come into balance in this way.

Elders, perhaps you have not been aware of the profound responsibility you are now to assume; if you had known you would have had the conscious opportunity to learn and deepen yourself in good relationships through your lifetime, that you might serve your people, that you might use yourself well in these years. Younger women, you who read this now, are conscious and can choose to learn and grow in this way, that you might feel ready when you, too, step into the Grandmother Lodge.

Among many of the tribes the primacy of the Law of Good Relationship was remembered and the Grandmother Lodges, or the societies within them, were known to hold the highest command. If a peace chief was not leading his. people across the land in a way that all people and animals had good food, clear water, and sheltering valleys in the time of cold winds, then the Grandmothers asked for someone new to lead; they called someone to step forth from the people who had the probability of doing a better job in his active work to nurture and renew the people. If a war chief was creating such animosity among surrounding tribes that frequent attacks disrupted the life and well-being of the people, he was asked to find productive rather than destructive uses for his energy. Such was their power: they took seriously the charge to nurture and renew the people, and took action in line with it.

As you begin gathering with others, you will likely have a small and mixed group, and need to determine the common interests, skills, and goals among you. Some of your time together may well be used to increase your own learning and understanding, meetings to share skills with each other, to meditate and to learn to listen to the Great Voices within, gatherings to hike upon the Earth or to strengthen and tone your bodies.

I am often asked about those of you who have experienced amenorrhea, early menopause, or hysterectomies: Where do you fit? My first thought is that you will very likely want to get a sense of the rhythm of the worldly Mystery that is your natural cycle which is synchronized with Grandmother Moon, for this cycle still echoes through the waters of your body, even though external Bleeding doesn't accompany it. Deepen your experience of the Moon's cycle within you and bring back vision for your people. Secondly, many of us who are younger and don't experience ourselves as Elders are being called into the Grandmother Lodge because there is an urgent need for the awakening of this function among women. Because of the crushing of the Native cultures, and the loss of the women's ways, there are few who sit in these Lodges upholding the nurturing and renewing of the people. So the younger, awakened of us are being called into the Lodge through many different means. Accept it as an honour.

The final aspect of the Grandmother Lodge I will address is the rite of passage into it. Those of you surrounding a woman who is crossing this threshold will want to honour this special woman and to let her know of your support for her. There are many ways this can be done: ritual bathing and anointing by a close friend; being dressed in a white gown (for wisdom) and a red sash (red to represent the '"Blood" or life force in All Our Relations and the dedication to them) for a circle dance and feasting; an honouring of her by each woman gathered expressing her appreciation for this woman; a special dedication from the honoured one can be given (such as I dedicate this portion of my life to the children of all generations, etc.). Certainly an invocation of the Goddess, of White Buffalo Woman, or the Wise Crone can be done, perhaps in the form of a guided meditation for the Elder one to deepen her contact with this source of strength and wisdom. You who know her will know those aspects which have special meaning for her. Always when I do such a ritual, I include as part of the rite, the charging of this woman with the primary responsibility of the nurturing and renewing of All Her Relations and remind her of Creator's Law of Good Relationship. Among you, one already in her Grandmother Lodge might perform this function.

And so I give away these thoughts to you, knowing that through your own experience you will deepen your knowing about them much beyond what I have spoken. Remember Mother Earth, Grandmother Moon, and Father Spirit live within you. Reach deep within your true nature and bring forth beauty!

❧

HYSTERECTOMY, AN ARTIFICIAL Rite of Passage, Cornwoman

Some women who have had hysterectomies feel left out when Moon circles and menstruation are discussed. To such women I say that I believe there is a place in the Moon Lodge for them if they choose it. A woman doesn't lose her spiritual womb just because her physical womb has been removed. The spiritual body cycle is still there, and by timing her physical activities according to the moon's phases, she can gain a lot of healing benefits and spiritual growth. For such women there may be many unresolved issues surrounding her operation. Joining a Moon Circle may help bring such issues into the open so that the healing process can take place. Every woman who loses her uterus and other female organs must, at some time, acknowledge that loss and go through the grieving process.

Looking at it from another point of view, a woman who has had a hysterectomy is blessed with two choices. She can stay in the Moon Lodge to understand her cycle better and work on healing and family issues, or, if she honestly feels that her Bleeding time is over, then joining the older women's circle or crone's lodge may be right for her. This would also mean that she accept the responsibilities of the crones to the best of her ability. As a woman who holds onto her Blood, she dedicates herself to work for the good of her community and the world.

Many women are having hysterectomies these days. This is sad because many times other kinds of medicine can be effective. Perhaps this awful situation causes some good if, as their family responsibilities lessen, these women feel called upon to devote their energies to the health of this planet.

⚜

C.N.S., TEACHER IN her late 40's; Victoria, BC

I had a lot of trouble with PMS all the time I was menstruating. After a pregnancy in which I lost the child at five-and-a-half months, I continued to Bleed sporadically and horrendously for six months. One time I was out with a friend and I started bleeding. Before we got home I had soaked the seat of her car. Another time when I went shopping alone, I started to Bleed and fainted. It got so bad, I couldn't go anywhere without carrying a grocery bag of pads with me. I hardly left the house. After six months, I decided to have a hysterectomy. I knew little about other alternatives; I just accepted what the doctors told me.

I knew nothing at all about alternative medicine. In later years I found that my problem was probably a ripped uterus and that the condition could have been cured by herbal remedies and exercises. After the operation, I was relieved to be rid of the problem, but later I went through a time of grieving, a time when I wished there had been some other way to solve my problem. Looking back, I realize I had only about fifteen years of menstruating before my operation. That is not a long time to Bleed. Later, I became involved in a relationship where I wanted to have a child, but couldn't. It wasn't a strong need, but it was there. At the same time it was a relief not to have to deal with the edema and other PMS symptoms I had experienced. I felt much more productive after my operation. Sometimes I was able to achieve a balance.

⚜

R.R., PSYCHOLOGIST in her 40's; New York, NY

Last year, a woman who had a hysterectomy came to me for counselling. The operation took place about five years before but, because of a new love relationship, a sense of grief and loss recently entered her consciousness. Over the weeks and months that followed, we talked a lot about why the operation happened and about her feelings, both then and now. Together we made time for her grieving process. What became clear to me was that this woman, like many other hysterectomy victims, only knew her body in a negative way. She was probably never taught to feel good about being a woman. Naturally, in these instances, the body, and especially the uterus, fights back with discomfort and pain. Women who don't enjoy being women are easy victims for unscrupulous doctors who want to cut out their womanhood.

This woman who came to me needed to let go, but along with that letting go and accepting the past, she needed to get in touch with her body in a positive way. I suggested some deep belly breathing techniques to connect her physical and spiritual centre. To help her focus on her centre (that point just below your navel the Japanese call the "hara"), I suggested she place a large crystal on her belly. In this way, she could breathe into her belly and the weight of the crystal would help her focus her energy there. This technique, in its many variations, is the key to a variety of spiritual disciplines around the world. It helps one to be in touch with the higher self, great spirit, the Goddess, or whatever one wishes to call the all knowing power.

After doing this breathing technique for a while, she seemed changed, and she admitted that she felt different; more at peace with herself.

Since that time, I recommend belly breathing to other women in my practice and to my personal friends. I've begun doing it regularly myself. It is a powerful tool. When I do this exercise, I feel a link through my centre to the centre of all things. I feel so alive. It is wonderful. In my work and my life-style in general, I tend to think about things, but I never really feel them deep down inside. I think it is important for us to get out of our "heads" and more into feeling with our "bellies." The world would be a better place if we did.

M., WITCH IN HER 50'S; rural BC

When my mother reached menopause, her physician advised a hysterectomy. She got a second opinion, which was the same as the first.

Both of these physicians were men. In spite of dire warnings, she decided against having the operation. The condition healed itself, and menopause progressed. She is now seventy-five and very healthy.

It is estimated that over seventy-five per cent of hysterectomies are unnecessary.

*

L.L., NURSE IN HER late 30's; Vancouver, BC

I had a hysterectomy a year ago. Before the operation, I was given little real information. My doctor claimed it would be the cure for everything wrong with me, from acne to depression. He was wrong and he also didn't tell me how dead I would feel inside. Before the hysterectomy, when my husband and I made love, my whole body would vibrate after orgasm. I felt so alive and that feeling came from deep inside my womb. This resonant feeling would last long after the orgasmic spasms had passed. Now, when we make love and I experience orgasm, it lasts for a moment and then it's gone. The uterus is gone and the feeling is flat and dead. There is no resonance, no vibration. Only deadness. Why couldn't they have told me about this awful emptiness before I agreed to have it done?

*

B.R., HEALTH CARE WORKER in her late 30's; Baltimore, MD

I work with severely disabled people and it disturbs me to see how these people, especially the women, are treated by the staff and doctors. It's standard practice to perform hysterectomies on severely retarded or disabled girls, sometimes even before they have their first period. I guess the doctors think they are doing the girls a favour. The staff won't have to deal with the mess, and the young women won't be frightened by the blood or get pregnant. I have such mixed feelings about this issue. Just because they can't talk so many disabled people are treated like animals or worse. From my own experience I know they can communicate in other ways, and they understand much more than people give them credit for. I wonder how an autistic young girl feels when she has her period, and how it feels to have an operation to remove all that. It's a difficult question. What are women's basic rights concerning their bodies?

⁓⁓⁓

M.L.B., IN HER 40'S; Halifax, NS

Ten years ago, I was in a car accident that paralyzed my legs. At the time, I had two or three operations to reverse the damage, but nothing worked. After my last hospital stay, I had no more periods. At first I thought it was the trauma of the accident. When the periods hadn't returned after a year, I asked my doctor if something was wrong with me. He then told me he removed my uterus during one of the operations.

I couldn't believe it because neither my husband nor I signed any papers. The doctor hadn't even talked to me about it. When I asked him why he did this he said he thought he was doing me a favour. Sitting in that chair all the time, he reasoned, I shouldn't have to put up with the mess each month. I was completely devastated and broke down right there. I had always wanted a baby. There wasn't anything wrong with me that way, and being in a wheelchair didn't mean I couldn't be a mother.

That damn doctor took it upon himself to play God and mess up my life. When I told my husband, he was very angry, but after a while he cooled down because he felt the damage had been done and there was nothing that we could do. If I had known then what I know now, I would have sued that doctor for every penny he had, told the press, and gotten some disabled activist groups to back me. My marriage broke up a year later, and, although he denies it, I've always felt my husband did not leave me because I was disabled, but because he wanted a woman who could give him a son.

⁓⁓⁓

L.B., GRANDMOTHER IN her early 50's; Northern Manitoba

I am from a small Indian reserve in Northern Canada. An old doctor used to work on our reserve who was doing some pretty awful things to some of the women there. It took a while for people to realize that there weren't as many babies being born after that doctor came. Eventually we discovered that, if a woman came to him with a problem that required hospitalization, he'd take out her uterus or tie her tubes while he performed whatever operation was actually needed. I know this for a fact because my aunt was one of the women he operated on. Later, he told her she'd gone through a premature menopause at forty-four. When the story came out, the Band was pretty mad about it, but the government transferred that doctor before the Band could do anything. I sometimes wonder where that old doctor is, and if he's still treating Native women on some other reserve the same way.

⚬⚬⚬

A HEALING RITUAL AFTER the Operation,

S.B., chinese medicine practitioner in her 40's; Vancouver Island, BC

Over a long period of time, I had gradually worsening problems with my menstrual cycles. I bled between periods and hemorrhaged a lot. Just before my operation, it seemed as if my period lasted about three weeks out of every month. The doctor tried a D&C, but that didn't seem to help. Next, he told me to go on the pill, but I didn't because of the bad side effects I experienced. I had a hormonal imbalance where the progesterone level never went down, and my uterus was swollen all the time. I was referred to a specialist who suggested getting rid of the problem. Life without periods would be so much easier and more pleasant, he said, and, besides, my uterus was useless now, right? In my ignorance, I thought it would be okay so he scheduled me for surgery. This doctor told me that a hysterectomy would cure many of my other health problems, including acne and sinus problems. I'd be in perfect health after I had the surgery because this female stuff was causing all my problems. I trusted him and went for it, thinking there'd be no problem. I didn't want any more children and was quite happy not to become pregnant again. I didn't anticipate any emotional reaction to the whole thing.

It was interesting what actually happened. Physically, I recovered quite quickly, but for a long time afterwards, I felt extremely fragile and emotionally quite vulnerable. I experienced much sadness and the doctor couldn't seem to tell me what was going on. He was also wrong about the operation curing all my other problems. They were still there, and I still experienced PMS.

On the advice of a couple of friends, I decided to have a ritual and say goodbye to that part of me. I started planning my ritual. I decided I would find something to represent my uterus. Ideally, it would have been wonderful to have my uterus itself, but that wasn't possible so I looked for a suitable replacement. A pomegranate would have been perfect, but since they were out of season, I chose an eggplant. For some reason, that looked like a womb to me. I don't know why, it just felt right. Late at night, I went to a special place in the woods with a friend. I set up candles for the four directions and created a circle. Then, I talked about my uterus and how I felt about it and what it had done for me. I talked about the joy of having my children.

As part of this ritual, I brought flowers that I felt represented my children. I don't remember exactly what flowers I chose, but I picked them according to their personalities. I had a bunch for each of my children. I thanked my uterus for each of them and spread the flowers in the woods. Then, I came back to the circle, dug a hole in the earth, and said goodbye to my uterus as I buried the eggplant. My friend and I had wine and cakes to celebrate. This was a very emotional experience for me. I cried a lot and was both sad and joyful at the same time.

After the ritual, I recovered my emotional balance. The ritual seemed to be a wonderful release for me. I certainly recommend this to anyone who loses a part of her body. I also recommend that surgery be the very last resort for anyone. Knowing what I know now, I would never have had a hysterectomy. I would have gotten acupuncture or herbal treatments instead. That was the last time I ever trusted a western doctor.

Now, I know my problem was due to an energy imbalance and a nutritional deficiency. If these health problems had been corrected, my uterus could have functioned quite normally. As it is, I have to deal with scar tissue and a lot of cramping when I ovulate. It's just not a natural state that I find myself in, and I'm wondering what repercussions I will have when I go through menopause. I am still very angry toward that specialist (male, of course!) who talked about how useless a uterus was after it has borne children. I'm deeply saddened that I was taught to be ashamed of having my period while I was growing up. I felt dirty then and I really worked hard not to instill that feeling in my children.

K.J., NURSE AND MIDWIFE in her 40's; Portland, OR

This June was the third anniversary of my living without my uterus. In a recent ritual, when M.G. talked about wounding, it touched my heart because most of the time when I go to women's gatherings, we talk about womb power, the menstrual hut, and about our Bloods being our time of power. I feel very hurt and excluded in these conversations and there is an aching and a longing within me that is hard to ignore. I feel as if I gave away my power before I even knew about it. At these gatherings, I feel invisible. I'm not a crone, I didn't go through a natural menopause, and I'm not a maiden, nor a Bleeding woman. Where do I fit in? I feel excluded, and there is a rage in me because I don't want to feel powerless and left out. My source of power still feels very visceral, very pelvic. I often forget that I don't have a uterus anymore.

When M.G. talked about hysterectomies as a type of wounding, and that all women have been wounded, I finally felt a part of the circle.

At the time of my hysterectomy three years ago, it didn't feel like a wounding. I had my tubes tied earlier, and I got what is called post-tubal ligation syndrome. Before my tubes were tied, I never had pain with my Bleeding, but after the tubal, it got worse until two weeks out of each month I was in agony – couldn't work, couldn't do anything.

My doctor, who was also my boss, told me that a hysterectomy was the only solution. I had tried herbal remedies with little success, and it was everyone's opinion that a hysterectomy was the only solution. My mother, who was visiting me at the time, said she wanted me to do it right then. I figured it would be impossible to arrange for a hysterectomy in three days – major surgery with a specific doctor, room and time – but my doctor got on the phone, and everything was arranged. At the time, it felt as if this operation was meant to happen.

I took my uterus home with me. I knew that, in the hospital, it would be cut up and examined and I didn't want that. This was the part of my body that grew my children, and it was sacred to me, so I wanted to deal with it in the proper manner. When it was cut from my body, I asked my doctor to show her to me. I would have taken her right then, except I was too overwhelmed. Instead, when I was ready to leave the hospital, I went to pathology and asked for her. The doctor showed me that he had put her in a bag with the last of my menstrual Blood, and he showed me how he had only taken the tiniest amount of tissue to check for cancer cells. That the doctor had done what I asked amazed me. I took her home and kept her in the refrigerator. I would take her out and look at her ... this part of me that had grown my children. I was able to touch her to my face, and cry with her, and share her with my children. I was able to show them this uterus, so small, in which they grew to eight and a half pounds. I told them that this part of my body had held and nurtured them as they grew for nine months. It was very special to me.

I buried her in my backyard with a medicine wheel that I had created. A sequoia tree that was a very important part of my life grew there. I wanted to make more of a ritual of it, but I was only five days post-op, and my mother was afraid I would hurt myself. It was very important that I dig the hole myself and pour the last of my menstrual Blood into the Earth, and then, with my own hands, lay my uterus in the ground and cover her. I cried and cried and sang to the Mother. I had to acknowledge what an important thing this was for me. It is absolutely sacred for me to know that she became part of the Earth and that the forget-me-knots that I planted there thrive.

One year later, I attended a women's spirituality gathering where everyone was talking about womb power and I felt horrible. Afterwards, I talked to my lover about how my heart felt broken being with other women and not feeling a part of the circle. My lover was convinced that we could do a healing circle for all women who had lost their femaleness to medical science. The circle was incredible. Out of three hundred women at that gathering, two-thirds of us were in the inner circle enfolded by the others. We held each other close and cried and cried. Everybody had tears running down their faces. It was so cleansing. In the past two years, I've gone to other healing circles which have helped. When M.G. talked about some of us being chosen to become crones early, to help with the healing of our earth, it was renewing for me to hear.

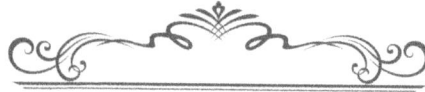

Appendix

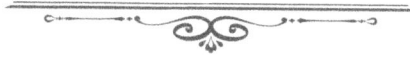

A Journey to the Moon Lodge

Included here is a guided visualization I often use in women's groups. It is a very powerful trigger which enables many women to get in touch with their feelings about menstruation and to openly talk about their periods for the first time.

It is my hope that houses like the one described here will one day be a part of all women's lives. This is my dream for the future.

Imagine, for a moment, that in some city or town there exists a sanctuary where women go to rest and renew their energies while Bleeding. In our minds anything is possible, so let us pay a visit to that wonderful house of healing and love we will call the Moon Lodge. Sit back, relax, and go to that imaginary place.

The lodge is a large, old house; its location could be on any quiet residential street in any city or town of our choosing. Surrounding the house is a beautiful, well-maintained garden and lawn. In the centre of that luxurious lawn is a brightly painted sign. In large letters across the top is written "Moon Lodge." Below are the words, "Menstrual Sanctuary – For Women Only." On the porch, two elderly women step out to welcome us. One has wise eyes and a warm smile. She explains that she and her companion are the caretakers of the Moon Lodge. She hopes our stay in the lodge will be a pleasant one. Let us go in.

These two elderly priestesses (for surely they are that) function as counsellors, house mothers, ceremonial leaders, and general keepers of the grounds. As we admire the house from the front hallway, our elderly guide explains that this house is owned and operated by women, for women. Many women who believe in what the lodge stands for contribute financially towards the maintenance of the house and the small salary paid its caretakers.

No money is accepted from men or institutions or companies run by men. In short, no government funding or interference is sought or accepted. In the past there have been hard times no doubt, but the Moon Lodge has weathered them because it has something uniquely special to offer women. Our guides invite us to take a tour of the house. We will begin by going upstairs.

As we climb, the melodic tones of wind chimes reach our ears from somewhere in the house. For just a moment, we stop to savour its lovely sound. Upstairs there are several large, airy bedrooms and a bath. Several healthy house plants act as accents to the deep, rich colours of the carpets and drapes. The smell of rose incense is in the air.

The bedrooms are furnished simply: a dresser, a small altar table with red candles always lit. Several foam pads or futons with red quilts are laid out on the floor. There are big, fluffy pillows scattered about for comfort, and a bookshelf in the hall should someone wish to read. Our guide explains quietly that these rooms are set aside for women wishing to rest, read quietly, or meditate. Socializing takes place in other parts of the house. Up here, silence is to be maintained as much as possible.

An atmosphere of peace and reverence embraces us like a mother welcoming home a long lost child. It would be nice to sit on one of the pallets, breathe in the incense, and melt into the silence and the candle flames. It would be nice, but our guide is gesturing for us to follow her back downstairs. There is much more to see, and these rooms are here anytime we might wish to return.

Downstairs, towards the front of the house, we are shown our guides' living quarters. Next to these rooms there is a large room that is used for the many classes taught here. Our guides explain that the Moon Lodge offers classes to women on a variety of subjects. Some of the most popular include menstruation and sex education for teens, childbirth, herbal medicine, and massage. This particular room is also available (for a small fee) to women's groups wishing to hold meetings in the lodge. Next to the classroom is the office and a smaller room that serves a variety of functions including counselling, massage, and emergency daycare for women attending classes in the larger room.

On the other side of the hall, we are shown a ceremonial room. This room was created by renovating several smaller rooms into one large room that runs almost the entire length of the house. In this room, the Moon rituals and other ceremonies are held. It is spacious enough to hold twenty or thirty women comfortably. The room is unfurnished, save for the brightly coloured pillows against the walls. There is a fireplace in the South and an elaborate altar table against the North wall. The drapes in this room are drawn, except towards the West where large glass doors open out onto the backyard garden. Above the doors we see the large wind chime that is the source of the lovely sounds heard throughout the house. The smell of incense and flowers mingle richly in the air. We step out into the garden. Because we are in an urban area, and as much privacy as possible is desired, the fence is high and covered with green. Towards the back is a vegetable garden and a few dwarf fruit trees. Near the house is an old oak and, at its base, a small fountain has been installed. Tiny, golden carp play in the depths of the fountain pool. There are flowers everywhere, especially roses.

Everything grows so well here, our guides explain, because many women who stay at the Moon Lodge offer the gift of their Blood to the Earth and the plants. It would be nice to pause here in this lovely garden in the sun, but once more, we must move on, saving further exploration until later.

Back in the ceremonial room we pause by the altar. A beautiful statue of the Goddess dominates the table. To either side of Her there are two red glass candles that are kept ever lit. To Her left sits a vase of red roses, and to Her right, a large red glass goblet for the ritual drink. At Her feet is an offering of incense and a shell filled with Moon Blood. In this room the sense of power and love are very strong; truly it has the feel of a sacred space. Gazing at the altar, an old longing, present yet unfocused, awakens once again within our hearts. Out there, in our world, there is loneliness, emptiness, guilt, and self-hatred. Our hearts hunger for the ancient wisdom that is our birthright, but that has been lost to so many of us. We thirst for love and acceptance and spiritual growth, and here at the feet of the Goddess, in this house, there is the hope that at last, our thirst will be quenched and our hunger satiated.

Our guides step close, offering us comfort with their physical presence and their words. They tell us that tonight there will be a Moon ritual held in this room and we are welcome to stay and participate. Tonight many women will tell their stories and share their wisdom with us. If we choose, we can take these teachings with us when we return to our world to comfort us and help us create our own Moon Lodges, wherever we are.

The sun is sinking towards the horizon and our guides invite us to come to the kitchen for tea and the evening meal. We accept gladly. In the Moon Lodge, the kitchen is the area for socializing. It is a large, old country style kitchen, furnished with a large oak table, a long comfortable couch, and a rocking chair. A combination wood and propane stove adds warmth and spirit to the place. To the left is a pantry filled with herbs and good but simple foods. The air is sweet with the smells of baking bread, herbs, and homemade soup bubbling on the stove. This room is warm and comfortable and always filled with the happy laughter of women. The kitchen of the Moon Lodge acts as a drop-in centre for women in the community. Any woman is welcome to come in, have some tea, and visit for a while. This room is bright, cheerful, and well used.

Over steaming cups of herb tea, our guide explains how the Moon Lodge is run. If a woman is having her period and feels a need to get away from her regular routine, she can call the Moon Lodge and ask to stay from one to five nights within any month. Women are asked to donate money (what they can afford), food, or some sort of service such as gardening, laundry, typing, or housework in exchange for their stay at the Lodge.

Because this is a "retreat" for women, children are discouraged from staying at the house. Breastfed babies may accompany their mothers, but toddlers and older children are not permitted to stay overnight. Children may visit with mothers for tea in the kitchen, but they aren't allowed upstairs. When a woman with small children wishes to stay at the Moon Lodge, she may check the babysitting list and either pay for a sitter, or trade off with another woman in a similar situation. The system has its ups and downs but, on the whole, functions quite well. No men are allowed in the house; even repairs are done by women. No drugs or alcohol are allowed in the house. Smoking is also discouraged and allowed only on the front porch or in part of the back garden.

We want a safe space here, one guide explains, a space where women can explore the rhythms of their bodies and spiritually heal and grow. This cannot be accomplished in an atmosphere of alcohol and drugs.

The sun has set and it grows late. We finish our meal and gather in the hallway with the other women waiting quietly for the ritual to begin. Beside the doorway, in the northeast, is a table on which a pitcher of water, basin, and incense burner lie. We come forward singly, smudge ourselves with sage, then pour water over our hands and face to ritually cleanse ourselves in preparation for the ceremony. After our ritual cleansing, we pass into the room clockwise, beginning in the East. A small altar has been set up in each of the directions to honour the four quarters. The larger altar we noticed before has been moved to the centre of the room. We walk around the room and pause for a moment at each to consider the Four Elements and their meaning in our lives.

In the East, the altar cloths are yellow and pale green. The element is air; the realm of mind and communication is honoured here. We ask ourselves:

How do I communicate with others? Do I see clearly through the illusions of things to inner truth?

We pass on to the fires of the South. A fire burns in the fireplace and above, on the mantle, red and orange cloths hang. Here the spark of life is kindled and the energies of our passions burst forth. We ask ourselves:

How am I using my energies? What attracts my passions? Are they of benefit to me or destroying me?

Next we pass near the open glass door to the altar of the West. Its colour is blue for the waters of life. In the garden the fountain sings softly. We are invited to touch some of the water in the cup to our foreheads in honour of life and love. We ask ourselves:

Where do my emotions flow? Can I plunge deep within to look at my inner feelings?

In the North is the element of Earth, cornerstone of all power. The altar colours are hues of green, brown, and black, the colours-of Earth, Herself. We pick up some soil from a bowl, and as it sifts back through our fingers, we ask ourselves:

Am I taking care of my body and my material needs well? Am I open to the power of the Earth and working to help Her survive?

When we have completed the circle we pass into the centre and sit quietly, waiting for the others to assemble. It is time to begin. Our two elderly guides step forward, transformed by their ritual robes from the kindly

grandmotherly women of the afternoon, to the priestesses of majesty and
power that they are.

The circle is formally opened by a ritual chant as the priestesses pass
around the circle four times. First by athalme and censer, then by fire, then
by water, then by blessed cornmeal is the circle cast. We now are between the
worlds, in sacred space. Outside the door, a dragon woman sits. Her job is to
make sure that, from this point on, no interruption will mar the rite.

The priestesses approach the centre altar. The invocation to the Goddess
is chanted. The room is filled with the power of the Great Mother. The drum
beats. We sing and dance, lifting up our hearts in gladness, forever thankful
for our many gifts, and for being who we are. It is so good to sing and move
our bodies in sacred dance. It is so good to be alive!

As the energy ebbs, we sit once more. The sacred cup is passed so that we
may drink of the wine (Moon Blood) of the Goddess. We sit, eyes shining,
smiling at the women around us. One of the priestesses holds up a carved
stick with deer hooves hanging from it. She shakes it for silence and our
attention. She begins to speak.

*In this Moon Lodge on this sacred day of the Moon, we have come together
to honour the Goddess within us and share our wisdom and our love with our
sisters. I offer you the talking stick carved with the serpent of the ancient wisdom.
Let us pass around the talking stick and share our stories and teachings so that as
in the old days, our woman's wisdom can be shared and passed on. By the power
of the Goddess, so it must be.*

And so, the stick is passed and stories told.

[At this point I have various women in the group read portions from
the main text of this book. These readings represent the stories being told by
the imaginary women in the Moon Lodge. I gather these stories from several
chapters and themes, thus creating a variety of pieces for women to identify
with and discuss later. After readings and any further discussions, I continue
with the guided visualization.]

The candles flicker and dim. It grows late. In that quiet hour just before
dawn, we sit quietly in the ceremonial room of the Moon Lodge. The talking
stick has been passed around the circle many times during the night as the
women share their stories and wisdom with us. Now it is late and all that
needed to be shared has been expressed. The night has been filled with

laughter and tears, joy and pain. The women of the Moon Lodge have given us a great gift which we can bring home with us to remember and savour often in times to come. It is time; the old priestess stands and, facing the centre altar, she gives thanks to the Goddess and bids Her farewell. Then facing each of the four candle points she addresses the guardians of the elements saying:

Powers of the Earth and water, powers of fire and air, in love we have summoned you, in love we release you and bid you farewell. The circle is open yet unbroken and may the peace of the Goddess be in your hearts always.

The candles are snuffed out as we leave the room in silence. Through the glass doors we can see the garden dimly in the pale light – dawn is very near. We stand once more on the porch of the Moon Lodge in the chill morning air. The women smile warmly at us as they pass by on their way home to bed and rest.

It's late and we are tired, but a wonderful feeling of contentment possesses our spirit as well. Wrapped in shawls, our guides come out to wish us farewell. We thank them for all they have shared with us. They smile and invite us to come back another time. We wave goodbye and then their image fades as drifting down through the mists we return to our own place and time. Breathe deep now and look around. Feel the solidity of the space around you. You are grounded and secure. We have come home.

This visit to the Moon Lodge has been a wonderful experience to imagine, and you can use that meditation to return to the Moon Lodge anytime you need a place where you can find peace and guidance in your life. Perhaps in the concrete reality of our day-to-day lives it would be nice to have a real menstrual sanctuary to visit now and then.

In many parts of Canada and the United States and elsewhere around the world, women are gathering in spiritual healing circles each Moon time to explore their own inner healing and spiritual growth. These circles are a beginning. They bring women together to talk and share their experiences as they honour the moon and the Goddess within.

As these circles deepen and stabilize, these women will also become aware of a need for stable gathering places in which to meet – a place that belongs to the group as a whole rather than any one member. This would be a place set aside as a sanctuary, a place to come to for individual meditation as well as group rituals.

For most groups a sanctuary in this form isn't possible right now, but through the medium of this book the idea has been magically made manifest in our world. Women's sanctuaries and places of learning are desperately needed for the women and girls of our time. It is my dream and fondest wish that by reading this book, you will be inspired to create in some form the reality of the Moon Lodge in your community. It is in this way that we can recapture the ancient teachings and pass on to our daughters the things we missed in our own lives. The Moon Lodge is the seed of a new beginning for women, for all humanity, and for the living Earth, Herself.

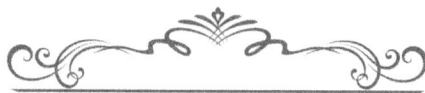

Bibliography

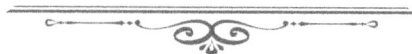

Women's Spirituality

Adler, Margo. *Drawing Down the Moon: Witches, Druids, Goddess-Worshippers and Other Pagans in America Today*. Boston, MA: Beacon Press, 1979.

Bolen, M.D., and Jean Shinoda. *Goddesses in Every Woman*. San Francisco, CA: Harper & Row, 1985.

Brinton, Perera, Sylvia. D*escent of the Goddess: Way of Initiation for Women*. Toronto, ON: Inner City Press, 1981.

Eisler, Riane. *The Chalice and the Blade: Our History, Our Future*. San Francisco, CA: Harper& Row, 1987.

Grahn, Judy. *Another Mother Tongue: Gay Words, Gay Worlds*. Boston, MA: Beacon Press, 1984.

Harding, M. Esther. *Woman's Mysteries Ancient and Modern*. New York, NY: Harper & Row. 1971.

Jamal, Michele. *Shapeshifters: Shaman Women in Contemporary Society*. New York, NY: Arkana, 1987.

Starhawk. *The Spiral Dance: A Rebirth of the Ancient Religion of the Great Goddess*. San Francisco, CA: Harper & Row, 1979.

Starhawk. *Dreaming in the Dark: Magic, Sex, and Politics*. Boston, MA: Beacon Press, 1982.

Stone, Merlin. *Ancient Mirrors of Womanhood*. Boston, MA: Beacon Press, 1979.

Teish, Luisah. J*ambalaya: The Natural Women's Book of Personal Charms and Practical Rituals*. San Francisco, CA: Harper & Row, 1985.

Walker, Barbara. *The Women's Encyclopedia of Myths and Secrets*. San Francisco, CA: Harper &Row, 1983.

Walker, Barbara. T*he Crone Women of Age, Wisdom, and Power*. San Francisco, CA: Harper & Row, 1985.

Weinstein, Marion. *Positive Magic: Occult Self-Help*. Washington, DC: Phoenix Publishing Inc., 1978.

Paths of Self-Awareness

Adair, Margot. *Working Inside Out: Tools for Change*. Berkeley, CA: Bookpeople, 1984.

Ashcroft-Nowicki, Dolores. *The Shining Paths: An Experiential Journey Through the Tree of Life*. Northamptonshire, UK: 1983.

Burka, Christa. *Clearing Crystal Consciousness*. Br. Life Inc, 1986.

Chia, Maneewan & Chia, Mantak. *Healing Love Through the Tao: Cultivating Female Sexual Energy*. New York, NY: Healing Tao Books, 2005.

Gardner, Joy. *Color and Crystals: A Journey Through the Chakras*. Freedom, CA: Crossing Press, 1987.

Gaskin, Ina May. *Spiritual Midwifery*. Summertown, IN: The Book Publishing Company, 1980.

Gordon, Richard. *Your Healing Hands: The Polarity Experience.* Mill Valley, CA: Orenda Unity Press, 1978.

Green, Marion. *The Path Through the Labyrinth: The Quest for Initiation into the Western Mystery Tradition.* Dorset, UK: Element Books, 1988.

Greer, Mary. *Tarot for Yourself: A Workbook for Personal Transformation.* North Hollywood, CA: Newcastle Publishing, 1984.

Greer, Mary. *Tarot Mirrors Reflections of Personal Meaning.* North Hollywood, CA: Newcastle Publishing, 1988.

Hay, Louise. *You Can Heal Your Life.* Santa Monica, CA: Hay House, 1984.

King, Serge. *Mastering Your Hidden Self: A Guide to the Huna Way.* Wheaton, IL: The Theosophical Publishing House, 1985.

Kirschmann, John D. *Nutrition Almanac.* New York, NY: McGraw Hill, 1984.

Lowen, Alexander M.D. & Lowen, Leslie. *The Way to Vibrant Health: A Manual of Bioenergetic Exercises.* New York, NY: Harper & Row, 1977.

Mariechild, Dianne. *Mother Wit: A Feminist Guide to Psychic Development.* New York, NY: Crossing Press, 1981.

Mindell, Arnold. *Working With the Dreambody.* New York, NY: Routledge & Kegan Paul, 1985.

Mindell, Arnold. *River's Way: The Process Science of the Dreambody.* New York, NY: Routledge & Kegan Paul, 1985.

Noble, Vicki. *Motherpeace: A Way to the Goddess through Myth, Art, and Tarot.* New York, NY: Harper & Row, 1983.

Pshashi, Wataru. *Do It Yourself Shiatsu.* New York, NY: E.D. Dutton, 1976.

Raphael, Katrina. *Crystal Enlightenment: The Transforming Properties of Crystals and Healing Stones.* New York, NY: Aurora Press, 1985.

Stein, Diana. *The Women's Book of Healing.* St. Paul, MN: Llewellyn, 1987.

Stein, Diana. *The Kwan Yin Book of Changes.* St. Paul, MN: Llewellyn, 1986.

Teeguarden, Iona Marsaa. *Acupressure Way of Health: Jin Sshin Do.* Tokyo, Japan: Japan Publications Inc, 1978.

Walker, Barbara. *The Secrets of the Tarot.* New York, NY: Harper & Row, 1984.

Aspects of Bleeding

Golub, Sharon. *Lifting the Curse of Menstruation: A Feminist Appraisal of the Influence of Menstruation on Women's Lives.* New York, NY: Harrington Park Press, 1985.

Kolkmeyer, Alexander. *The Clear Red Stone: A Myth and the Meaning of Menstruation.* Santa Fe, NM: In Sight Press, 1982. (A coming of age story for young women.)

Lander, Louise. *Images of Bleeding: Menstruation as Ideology.* New York, NY: Orlando Press, 1988.

Larks, Dr. Susan. *Premenstrual Syndrome Self-Help Book.* Los Angeles, CA: Forman Publishing, 1984.

Nazzaro, Dr. Ann & Lombard, Dr Donald. The PMS Solution: The Nutritional Approach. London: Eden Press, 1985.

Shuttle, Penelope & Redgrove, Peter. *The Wise Wound*. London, UK: Grafton Books, 1986.

Herbs

Beyerl, Paul. *The Master Book of Herbalism*. Washington, DC: Phoenix Publishing Co., 1984.

Cunningham, Scott. *Magical Herbalism*. St Paul, MN: Llewellyn Publications, 1983.

Grieve, Mrs M. *A Modern Herbal*. Volume 1 & 2. New York, NY: Dover Publications Inc, 1971.

Hoffmann, David. *The Holistic Herbal*. Findhorn, UK: Findhorn Press, 1983.

Jackson, Mildred & Teague, Terri. *The Handbook of Alternatives to Chemical Medicine*. Berkeley, CA: Bookpeople, 1983.

Potts, Billie. *Witches Heal Lesbian Herbal Self-Sufficiency*. New York, NY: Hecuba's Daughters Inc., 1981.

Tierra, Michael. *The Way of Herbs*. New York, NY: Washington Square Press, 1983.

Weed, Susan. *For the Childbearing Year*. New York, NY: Ash Tree Publishing, 1986.

Weed, Susan. *Healing Wise*. New York, NY: Ash Tree Publishing, 1989.

Miscellaneous

Leonard, Jim & Laut, Phil. *Rebirthing: The Science of Enjoying All of Your Life*. Cincinnati, OH: Trinity Press, 1983.

Orbach, Susie. *Fat is a Feminist Issue*. New York, NY: Berkley Books, 1982.

Reitz, Rosetta. *Menopause: A Positive Approach*. New York, NY: Penguin Books, 1977.

Seidman, Maruti. *A Guide to Polarity Therapy: The Gentle Art of Hands-On Healing*. North Hollywood, CA: Newcastle, 1986.

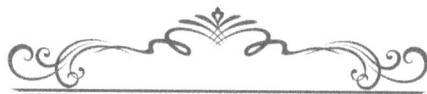

Acknowledgements

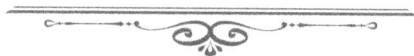

P. 37 "The Rite of Passage into Womanhood," De-Anna Alba, quoted from *Circle Network News* by permission of the author.

p. 40 "Blending Many Cultures in a Gift of Love," by Rachel Wallace, quoted with permission from I*n Context: A Quarterly of Humane Sustainable Culture*, P.O. Box 215, Sequim, WA, 98382.

p. 64 "A Menstrual Meditation," by Jean Mountaingrove, is available in *Women of Power*, Issue VIII.

p. 85 This quoted from *Womanspirit* (1974) with permission of the author.

p. 109 "The Blood Mystery: A Return to Our Shamanic Roots," by Vicki Noble, quoted by permission of the author.

p. 113 "Sacred Time, Sacred Way," by Brook Medicine Eagle, quoted by permission of the author.

p. 115 "The Women's Lodge," by Guaba Guarikgku, quoted by permission of the author.

p. 175 "Honouring Our Grandparents," by Spider, quoted by permission of the author.

p. 178 "Rites of Passage: Celebrating the Crone," by Maggie, quoted from *All My Relations* newsletter by permission of the author.

p. 180 Rainbow is taken from "Broomstick" by Emma Joy, editor of *A Web of Crones*.

Don't miss out!

Visit the website below and you can sign up to receive emails whenever Celu Amberstone publishes a new book. There's no charge and no obligation.

https://books2read.com/r/B-A-YGQM-WAVKB

BOOKS 2 READ

Connecting independent readers to independent writers.

Also by Celu Amberstone

Renewal
The Prophecy of Manu
Teoni's Giveaway

Rituals
Blessings of the Blood: A Book of Menstrual Lore and Rituals for Women
Deepening the Power: Community Ritual and Sacred Theatre

Tales of the Kashallans
The Dream-Chosen
The Hunted Kashallan
The Outlawed Bond
Uncertain Refuge
Prey of the Umwira
Blood Magic's Snare

Standalone
Refugees and Other Stories

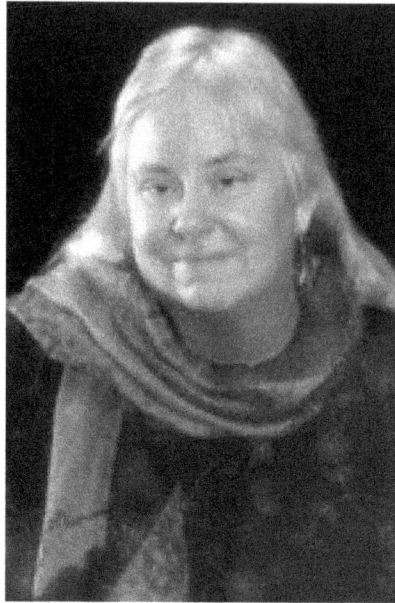

About the Author

Celu is of mixed Cherokee and Scots-Irish ancestry. Celu Amberstone was one of the few young people in her family to take an interest in learning Traditional Native crafts and medicine ways. This interest made several of the older members of her family very happy while annoying others.

Legally blind since birth, she has defied her limitations and spent much of her life avoiding cities. Moving to Canada after falling in love with a Métis-Cree man from Manitoba, she has lived in the rain forests of the west coast, a tepee in the desert and a small village in Canada's arctic. Along the way she also managed to acquire a BA in cultural anthropology and an MA in health education. Celu loves telling stories and reading. She lives in Victoria British Columbia near her grown children and grandchildren.

About the Publisher

Kashallan Press is an independent publisher releasing books by author Celu Amberstone. Among her books are critically-acclaimed works now re-released by Kashallan Press, and new works showcasing her talents in writing both fiction and non-fiction.

www.ingramcontent.com/pod-product-compliance
Lightning Source LLC
LaVergne TN
LVHW011324080426
835513LV00006B/186